Renal Diet Cookbook:

200+ Low-Sodium, Potassium, and Phosphorus Recipes for Your Kidney Disease. Learn how it is Easy to Avoid Dialysis and Optimize Your Health

SUSAN BUCKLEY

Table of Contents

Introduction

If you have been diagnosed with kidney dysfunction, a proper diet is necessary for controlling the amount of toxic waste in the bloodstream. When toxic waste piles up in the system along with increased fluid, chronic inflammation occurs and we have a much higher chance of developing cardiovascular, bone, metabolic or other health issues.

Since your kidneys can't fully get rid of waste on their own, which comes from food and drinks, probably the only natural way to help our system is through this diet.

A Renal Diet Is Especially Useful During the First Stages of Kidney Dysfunction and Leads to The Following Benefits:

- Prevents excess fluid and waste build-up

- prevents the progression of renal dysfunction stages

- Decreases the likelihood of developing other chronic health problems e.g. heart disorders

- has a mild antioxidant function in the body, which keeps inflammation and inflammatory responses under control.

The above-mentioned benefits are noticeable once the patient follows the diet for at least a month and then continuing it for longer periods, to avoid the stage where dialysis is needed. The strictness of the diet depends on the current stage of renal/kidney disease, if, for example, you are in the 3rd or 4th stage, you should follow a stricter diet and be attentive for the food, which is allowed or prohibited.

There is a distinct connection between the health and function of our kidneys and the way we eat. How we eat and the foods we choose make a significant impact on how well we feel and our overall well-being. Making changes to your diet is often necessary to guard against medical conditions, and while eating well can treat existing conditions, healthy food choices can also help prevent many other conditions from developing – including kidney disease.

When we make changes to our diet, we often focus on the restrictions or foods we should avoid. While this is important, it's also vital to learn about the foods and nutrients we need in order to maintain good health and prevent disease. Consider the related conditions that contribute to high blood pressure and type 2 diabetes, and the dietary changes often suggested to treat and, in some successful cases, reverse the damage of these conditions. Dietary changes for the treatment and prevention of disease often focus on limiting salt, sugar, and trans fats from our food choices, while increasing minerals, protein, and fiber, among other beneficial nutrients. The renal diet also focuses on eliminating, or at least limiting, the consumption of various ingredients to aid our kidneys to function better and to prevent further damage from occurring.

There are many foods that work well within the renal diet, and once you see the available variety, it will not seem as restrictive or difficult to follow. The key is focusing on the foods with a high level of nutrients, which make it easier for the kidneys to process waste by not adding too much that the body needs to discard. Balance is a major factor in maintaining and improving long-term renal function.

A lot of the recipes are fast and simple to make with common and relatively affordable ingredients. Appropriate serving suggestions are provided in many of the recipes. A practical information category includes tips to achieve success with this diet and a few ideas for snacks and meals. Also, I'm aware that a lot of people follow a restricted diet, desire to lose weight or maybe even have to gain weight. This is why I have come up with recipes that can be modified to meet your personal requirements.

If you have kidney failure, damaged kidney or symptoms of kidney problems then you must follow a renal diet. The renal diet focuses more on the foods you should avoid because they are directly detrimental to your kidney health.

The kidneys are fundamental organs for our life and they want an essential function for our health.

Following a balanced and correct diet is essential to preserve the health of the kidneys. However, there are some common risk factors that can affect the health of these organs. Diabetes and high blood pressure are at the top of the list of diseases that can damage the kidneys. Obesity, genetics and age can then increase the risk of getting kidney disease

Chapter 1: What you need to know about kidney disease

Before stepping further into the depths of the renal diet, let us learn more about our kidneys and how they function. This basic understanding can ensure a better awareness of kidney disease. Our kidneys act just like a filter; in fact, they are the natural filter of the body, which mainly filters the blood running into them with high pressure. There is one kidney on either side of the body; they both work in sync to clean and purify the entire body's blood constantly and consistently. The renal arteries that enter the kidneys also pass by the membranes in it, which only let the harmful excretory products to pass into the ureters of the kidneys and render the blood cleaned and purified. There is another vital function that the kidneys play which is to keep the water and electrolyte balance maintained in the body. If our body has water in excess, the kidneys will release it through urination, and if our body is dehydrated, then more water is retained. This smart mechanism is only possible when a critical mineral balance is maintained inside the kidney cells since the release of water can only occur through osmosis.

Kidney function or renal function are the terms used to explain how well the kidneys function. A healthy individual is born with a pair of kidneys. This is why whenever one of the kidneys lost its functioning it went unnoticed due to the function of the other kidney. But if the kidney functions further drop altogether and reach a level as low as 25 percent, it turns out to be serious for the patients. People who have only one kidney functioning need proper external therapy and in worst cases, a kidney transplant.

Kidney diseases occur when a number of renal cells known as nephrons are either partially or completely damaged and fail to filter blood entering in properly. The gradual damage of the kidney cells can occur due to various reasons, sometimes it is the acidic or toxic build-up inside the kidney over time, at times it is genetic, or the result of other kidney damaging diseases like hypertension (high blood pressure) or diabetes.

Chronic Kidney Disease (CKD)

CKD or chronic kidney disease is the stage of kidney damage where it fails to filter the blood properly. The term chronic is used to refer to gradual and long-term damage to an organ. Chronic kidney disease is therefore developed after a slow yet progressive damage to the kidneys. The symptoms of this disease only appear when the toxic wastes start to build up in the body. Therefore, such a stage should be prevented at all costs. Hence, early diagnosis of the disease proves to be significant. The sooner the patient realizes the gravity of the situation, the better measures he can take to curb the problem.

WHAT ARE THE CAUSES OF KIDNEY DISEASE?

There is never a single cause for a disease; a number of factors come into play and together become the source of the renal deficiency. As stated earlier, these causes may include the genetics of a person, some other health disorders that may damage the kidneys and the kind of lifestyle a person lives. The following are the most commonly known causes of renal disease.

- Heart disease

- Diabetes

- Hypertension (High blood pressure)

- Being around 60 years old

- Having kidney disease in family

SIGNS OF RENAL DISEASE

The good thing is that we can prevent the chronic stage of renal disease by identifying the early signs of any form of kidney damage. Even when a person feels minor changes in his body, he should consult an expert to confirm if it might lead to something serious. The following are a few of the early symptoms of renal damage:

- Tiredness or drowsiness

- Muscle cramps

- Loss of appetite

- Changes in the frequency of urination

- Swelling of hands and feet

- A feeling of itchiness

- Numbness

- The darkness of skin

- Trouble in sleeping

- Shortness of breath

- The feeling of nausea or vomiting

These symptoms can appear in combination with one another. These are general signs of body malfunction, and they should never be ignored. And if they are left unnoticed, they can lead to worsening of the condition and may appear as:

- Back pain

- Abdominal pain

- Fever

- Rash

- Diarrhea

- Nosebleeds

- Vomiting

After witnessing any of these symptoms, a person should immediately consult a health expert and prepare himself or herself for the required lifestyle changes.

Renal disease diagnostic tests

Besides identifying the symptoms of kidney disease, there are other better and more accurate ways to confirm the extent of loss of renal function. There are mainly two important diagnostic tests:

1. Urine test

The urine test clearly states all the renal problems. The urine is the waste product of the kidney. When there is loss of filtration or any hindrance to the kidneys, the urine sample will indicate it through the number of excretory products present in it. The severe stages of chronic disease show some amount of protein and blood in the urine. Do not rely on self-tests; visit an authentic clinic for these tests.

2. Blood pressure and blood test

Another good way to check for renal disease is to test the blood and its composition. A high amount of creatinine and other waste products in the blood clearly indicates that the kidneys are not functioning properly. Blood pressure can also be indicative of renal disease. When the water balance in the body is disturbed, it may cause high blood pressure. Hypertension can both be the cause and symptom of kidney disease and therefore should be taken seriously.

HOW TO KEEP YOUR KIDNEYS HEALTHY

Like all other parts of the body, human kidneys also need much care and attention to work effectively. It takes a few simple and consistent measures to keep them healthy. Remember that no medicine can guarantee good health, but only a better lifestyle can do so. Here are a few of the practices that can keep your kidneys stay healthy for life.

1. Active lifestyle

An active routine is imperative for good health. This may include regular exercise, yoga, or sports and physical activities. The more you move your body, the better its metabolism gets. The loss of water is compensated by drinking more water, and that constantly drains all the toxins and waste from the kidneys. It also helps in controlling blood pressure, cholesterol levels, and diabetes, which indirectly prevents kidney disease.

2. Control blood pressure

Constant high blood pressure may cause glomerular damage. It is one of the leading causes, and every 3 out of 5 people suffering from hypertension also suffer from kidney problems. The normal human blood pressure is below 120/80 mmHg. When there is a constant increase of this pressure up to 140/100mmHg or more it should be immediately put under control. This can be done by minimizing the salt intake, controlling the cholesterol level and taking care of cardiac health.

3. Hydration

Drinking more water and salt-free fluids proves to be the life support for kidneys. Water and fluids dilute the blood consistency and lead to more urination; this in turn will release most of the excretions out of the body without much difficulty. Drinking at least eight glasses of water in a day is essential. It is basically the lack of water which strains the kidneys and often hinders the glomerular filtration. Water is the best option, but fresh fruit juices with no salt and preservatives are also vital for kidney health. Keep all of them in constant daily use.

4. Dietary changes

There are certain food items which taken in excess can cause renal problems. In this regard, an extremely high protein diet, food rich in sodium, potassium, and phosphorous can be harmful. People who are suffering from early stages of renal disease should reduce their intake, whereas those facing critical stages of CKD should avoid their use altogether. A well-planned renal diet can prove to be significant in this regard. It effectively restricts all such food items from the diet and promotes the use of more fluids, water, organic fruits, and a low protein meal plan.

5. No smoking/alcohol

Smoking and excessive use of alcohol are other names for intoxication. Intoxication is another major cause of kidney disease, or at least it aggravates the condition. Smoking and drinking alcohol indirectly pollute the blood and body tissues, which leads to progressive kidney damage. Begin by gradually reducing alcohol consumption and smoking down to a minimum.

6. Monitor the changes

Since the early signs of kidney disease are hardly detectable, it is important to keep track of the changes you witness in your body. Even the frequency of urination and loss of appetite are good enough reasons to be cautious and concerning. It is true that only a health expert can accurately diagnose the disease, but personal care and attention to minor changes is of key importance when it comes to CKD.

Chapter 2: Five stages of kidney disease

THE FIVE STAGES OF KIDNEY DISEASE

Chronic kidney disease is categorized into five stages, each one characterized by a certain degree of damage done to the kidneys and rate of glomerular filtration, which is the rate at which filtration takes place in the kidneys. These help us understand just how well the kidneys are functioning.

Stage 1

The first stage is the least severe and actually comes close to a healthy state of your kidneys. Most people will never be aware if they have entered stage 1 of chronic kidney disease, or CKD. In many cases, if people discover stage 1 CKD, then it is because they were being tested for diabetes or high blood pressure. Otherwise, people can find out about stage 1 CKD if they discover protein or blood in the urine, signs of kidney damage in an ultrasound, a computerized tomography (CT) scan or through magnetic resonance imaging (MRI). If people have a family history of polycystic kidney disease (PKD), then there are chances that they might have CKD as well.

Stage 2

In this stage, there is a mild decrease in the glomerular filtration rate. People don't usually notice any symptoms at this stage as well. The reasons for discovering any signs of CKD is the same as with the reasons provided in stage 1.

So what's the difference between stage 1 and stage 2? It all lies in the glomerular filtration rate, or GFR for short. The GFR is measured in milliliters/minute.

In stage 1, the glomerular filtration rate (GFR) is around 90 ml/min. The normal range of the GFR is from 90 ml/min to 120 ml/min. So as you can see, stage 1 CKD shows a GFR at the lower end of the range. Because it falls so close to a normal rate, it easily goes unnoticed. At stage 2, the GFR falls to between 60-89 ml/min. You might become concerned with the range stage 2 falls in, but your kidneys are actually resilient. Even if they are not functioning at 100 percent, your kidneys are capable of doing a good job. So good that you might not notice anything was out of the ordinary.

Even though the differences between stage 1 and 2 are minuscule, they cannot be combined because the chances of someone showing certain symptoms of CKD when in stage 2 are greater.

Stage 3

At this stage, the kidneys suffer moderate damage. In order to properly gauge the level of damage, this stage is further divided into two: stage 3A and stage 3B. The reason for the division is because even though the severity of the disease worsens from 3A to 3B, the damage to the kidneys are still within moderate levels.

Each of the divisions are characterized by their GFR.

- 3A has a GFR between 45-59 ml/min

- 3B has a GFR between 30-44 ml/min

When patients reach stage 3, they begin to experience other symptoms of CKD, which include the below:

- Increase in fatigue

- Shortness of breath and swelling of extremities, also called edema

- Slight kidney pain, where the pain is felt in the lower back area

- Change in the color of urine

Stage 4

At stage 4, the kidney disease becomes severe. The GFR falls down to 15-30 ml/min. As the waste buildup increases the patient might experience nausea and vomiting, a buildup of urea in the blood that could cause bad breath, and find themselves having trouble doing everyday tasks such as reading a newspaper or trying to write up an email.

It is important to see a nephrologists' (a doctor who specializes in kidney problems) when the patient reaches stage 4.

Stage 5

At stage 5, the kidneys have a GFR of less than 15 ml/min. This is a truly low rate that causes the waste buildup to reach a critical point. The organs have reached an advanced stage CKD, causing them to lose almost all their abilities in order to function normally.

HOW TO PREVENT DIALYSIS NATURALLY

Dialysis steps in as a last case scenario when both kidneys lose sufficient function to clean the blood. Before the toxicity reaches a damaging level, it must be eradicated through external sources. Individuals who suffer from acute kidney diseases end up going through dialysis to get their blood cleaned through the artificial dialysis machine. This dialysis machine mimics the role of our kidneys, and the blood is pumped into the machine, and then it is pumped back into the body simultaneously. People who never went through dialysis should know that it is one long and exhaustive process, which every renal patient hates to go through. Fortunately, there are some effective measures to avoid dialysis. This precautionary measure can stop the progression of renal disease and even cure it to some extent.

- Exercise regularly

- Don't smoke

- Avoid excess salt in your diet

- Control of diabetes

- Eat correctly and lose excess weight

- Control high blood pressure

- Talk with your health care team

Chapter 3: Sodium, Potassium and Phosphorous roles in our body

SODIUM

Sodium is considered the most important electrolyte of the body next to chloride and potassium. The electrolytes are actually the substance that controls the flow of fluids into the cells and out of them. Sodium is mainly responsible for regulating blood volume and pressure. It is also involved in controlling muscle contraction and nerve functions. The acid-base balance in the blood and other body fluids is also regulated by sodium. Though sodium is important for the health and regulation of important body mechanisms, excessive sodium intake, especially when a person suffers from some stages of chronic kidney disease, can be dangerous. Excess sodium disrupts the critical fluid balance in the body and inside the kidneys. It then leads to high blood pressure, which in turn negatively affects the kidneys. Salt is one of the major sources of sodium in our diet, and it is strictly forbidden on the renal diet. High sodium intake can also lead to Edema, which is swelling of the face, hands, and legs. Furthermore, high blood pressure can stress the heart and cause the weakening of its muscles. The build-up of fluid in the lungs also leads to shortness of breath.

POTASSIUM

Potassium is another mineral that is closely linked to renal health. Potassium is another important electrolyte, so it maintains the fluid balance in the body and its pH levels as well. This electrolyte also plays an important role in controlling nerve impulses and muscular activity. It works in conjugation with the sodium to carry out all these functions. The normal potassium level in the blood must range between 3.5 and 5.5mEq/L. It is the kidneys that help maintain this balance, but without their proper function, the potassium starts to build up in the blood. Hyperkalemia is a condition characterized by high potassium levels. It usually occurs in people with chronic kidney disease. The prominent symptoms of high potassium are numbness, slow pulse rate, weakness, and nausea. Potassium is present in green vegetables and some fruits, and these ingredients should be avoided on a renal diet.

PHOSPHOROUS

The amount of phosphorus in the blood is largely linked to the functioning of the kidneys. Phosphorus, in combination with vitamin D, calcium, and parathyroid hormone, can regulate the renal function. The balance of phosphorous and calcium is maintained by the kidneys, and this balance keeps the bones and teeth healthy. Phosphorous, along with vitamin D, ensures the absorption of calcium into the bones and teeth, where this mineral is important for the body. On the other hand, it gets dangerous when the kidneys fail to control the amount of phosphorus in the blood. This may lead to heart and bone-related problems. Mainly there is a high risk of weakening of the bones followed by the hardening of the tissues due to the deposition of phosphorous and calcium outside the bones. This abnormal calcification can occur in the lungs, skin, joints, and arteries, which can become in time very painful. It may also result in bone pain and itching.

Chapter 4: What to eat and avoid in the renal diet

FOODS TO EAT

Many foods work well within the renal diet. Once you see the available variety, it will not seem as restrictive or difficult to follow. The key is focusing on the foods with a high level of nutrients, which make it easier for the kidneys to process waste by not adding too much that the body needs to discard. Balance is a major factor in maintaining and improving long-term renal function.

Garlic

An excellent, vitamin-rich food for the immune system, garlic is a tasty substitute for salt in a variety of dishes. It acts as a significant source of vitamin C and B6, while aiding the kidneys in ridding the body of unwanted toxins. It's a great, healthy way to add flavor for skillet meals, pasta, soups, and stews.

Berries

All berries are considered a good renal diet food due to their high level of fiber, antioxidants, and delicious taste, making them an easy option to include as a light snack or as an ingredient in smoothies, salads, and light desserts. Just one handful of blueberries can provide almost one day's vitamin C requirement, as well as a boost of fiber, which is good for weight loss and maintenance.

Bell Peppers

Flavorful and easy to enjoy both raw and cooked, bell peppers offer a good source of vitamin C, vitamin A, and fiber. Along with other kidney-friendly foods, they make the detoxification process much easier while boosting your body's nutrient level to prevent further health conditions and reduce existing deficiencies.

Onions

This nutritious and tasty vegetable is excellent as a companion to garlic in many dishes, or on its own. Like garlic, onions can provide flavor as an alternative to salt, and provides a good source of vitamin C, vitamin B, manganese, and fiber, as well. Adding just one quarter or half of an onion is often enough for most meals, because of its strong, pungent flavor.

Macadamia Nuts

If you enjoy nuts and seeds as snacks, you many soon learn that many contain high amounts of phosphorus and should be avoided or limited as much as possible. Fortunately, macadamia nuts are an easier option to digest and process, as they contain much lower amounts of phosphorus and make an excellent substitute for other nuts. They are a good source of other nutrients, as well, such as vitamin B, copper, manganese, iron, and healthy fats.

Pineapple

Unlike other fruits that are high in potassium, pineapple is an option that can be enjoyed more often than bananas and kiwis. Citrus fruits are generally high in potassium as well, so if you find yourself craving an orange or grapefruit, choose pineapple instead. In addition to providing a high levels of vitamin B and fiber, pineapples can reduce inflammation thanks to an enzyme called bromelain.

Mushrooms

In general, mushrooms are a safe, healthy option for the renal diet, especially the shiitake variety, which are high in nutrients such as selenium, vitamin B, and manganese. They contain a moderate amount of plant-based protein, which is easier for your body to digest and use than animal proteins. Shiitake and portobello mushrooms are often used in vegan diets as a meat substitute, due to their texture and pleasant flavor.

FOODS YOU NEED TO AVOID

Eating restrictions might be different depending upon your level of kidney disease. If you are in the early stages of kidney disease, you may have different restrictions as compared to those who are at the end-stage renal disease, or kidney failure. In contrast to this, people with an end-stage renal disease requiring dialysis will face different eating restrictions. Let's discuss some of the foods to avoid while being on the renal diet.

Dark-Colored Colas contain calories, sugar, phosphorus, etc. They contain phosphorus to enhance flavor, increase its life and avoid discoloration. Which can be found in a product's ingredient list. This addition of phosphorus varies depending on the type of cola. Mostly, the dark-colored colas contain 50–100 mg in a 200-ml serving. Therefore, dark colas should be avoided on a renal diet.

Avocados are a source of many nutritious characteristics plus their strong fats, fiber, and antioxidants. Individuals suffering from kidney disease should avoid them because they are rich in potassium. 150 grams of an avocado provides a whopping 727 mg of potassium. Therefore, avocados, including guacamole, must be avoided on a renal diet, especially if you are on a parole to watch your potassium intake.

Canned Foods including soups, vegetables, and beans, are low in cost but contain high amounts of sodium due to the addition of salt to increase its life. Due to this amount of sodium inclusion in canned goods, it is better that people with kidney disease should avoid consumption. opt for lower-sodium content with the label "no salt added". One more way is to drain or rinse canned foods, such as canned beans and tuna, could decrease the sodium content by 33–80%, depending on the product.

Brown Rice is a whole grain containing a higher concentration of potassium and phosphorus than its white rice counterpart. One cup already cooked brown rice possess about 150 mg of phosphorus and 154 mg of potassium, whereas, one cup of already cooked white rice has an amount of about 69 mg of phosphorus and 54 mg of potassium. Bulgur, buckwheat, pearled barley and couscous are equally beneficial, low-phosphorus options and might be a good alternative instead of brown rice.

Bananas are high potassium content, low in sodium, and provides 422 mg of potassium per banana. It might disturb your daily balanced potassium intake to 2,000 mg if a banana is a daily staple.

Whole-Wheat Bread may harm individuals with kidney disease. But for healthy individuals, it is recommended over refined, white flour bread. White bread is recommended instead of whole-wheat varieties for individuals with kidney disease just because it has phosphorus and potassium. If you add more bran and whole grains in the bread, then the amount of phosphorus and potassium contents goes higher.

Oranges and Orange Juice are enriched with vitamin C content and potassium. 184 grams provides 333 mg of potassium and 473 mg of potassium in one cup of orange juice. With these calculations, they must be avoided or used in a limited amount while being on a renal diet. Other alternatives for oranges and orange juice are apples, grapes and their cinder or juices as they possess low potassium contents.

Potatoes and sweet potatoes, being, the potassium-rich vegetables with 156 g contains 610 mg of potassium, whereas 114 g contains 541 mg of potassium which is relatively high. Some of the high-potassium foods, likewise potatoes and sweet potatoes, could also be soaked or leached to lessen the concentration of potassium contents. Cut them into small and thin pieces and boil those for at least 10 minutes can reduce the potassium content by about 50%. Potatoes which are soaked in a wide pot of water for as low as four hours before cooking could possess even less potassium content than those not soaked before cooking. This is known as "potassium leaching," or the "double cook Direction."

Snack foods like pretzels, chips, and crackers are the foods that lack in nutrients and are much higher in salt. It is very easy to take above the suggested portion, which lead to even greater salt intake than planned. If chips, being made from potatoes, they will contain a significant amount of potassium as well.

If you are suffering from or living with kidney disease, reducing your potassium, phosphorus and sodium intake is an essential aspect of managing and tackling the disease. The foods with high-potassium, high-sodium, and high-phosphorus content listed above should always be limited or avoided. These restrictions and nutrients intakes may differ depending on the level of damage to your kidneys. Following a renal diet might be a daunting procedure and a restrictive one most of the times. But, working with your physician and nutrition specialist and a renal dietitian can assist you to formulate a renal diet specific to your individual needs.

Chapter 5: 21-day meal plan

Days	Breakfast	Lunch	Dinner	Snacks
1	Egg White and Broccoli Omelette	Lemon & Herb Chicken Wraps	Vegetarian Gobi Curry	Edamame Guacamole
2	Yogurt Parfait with Strawberries	Ginger & Bean Sprout Steak Stir-Fry	Lemon Butter Salmon	Toasted Pear Chips
3	Eggs in Tortilla	Carrot & Ginger Chicken Noodles	Crab Cake	Citrus Sesame Cookies
4	American Blueberry Pancakes	Roast Beef	Baked Fish in Cream Sauce	Traditional Spritz Cookies
5	Raspberry Peach Breakfast Smoothie	Beef Brochettes	Shrimp & Broccoli	Classic Baking Powder Biscuits
6	Fast Microwave Egg Scramble	Country Fried Steak	Shrimp in Garlic Sauce	Crunchy Chicken Salad Wraps
7	Mango Lassi Smoothie	Beef Pot Roast	Fish Taco	Tasty Chicken Meatballs
8	Breakfast Maple Sausage	Meat Loaf	Baked Trout	Herb Roasted Cauliflower
9	Summer Veggie Omelet	Spiced Lamb Burgers	Spicy Veggie Pancakes	Sautéed Butternut Squash
10	Raspberry Overnight Porridge	Pork Loins with Leeks	Egg and Veggie Fajitas	German Braised Cabbage
11	Berry Chia with Yogurt	Chinese Beef Wraps	Vegetable Biryani	Walnut Pilaf
12	Arugula Eggs with Chili Peppers	Grilled Skirt Steak	Pesto Pasta Salad	Wild Mushroom Couscous
13	Breakfast Skillet	Spicy Lamb Curry	Barley Blueberry Avocado Salad	Basic Meat Loaf
14	Eggs in Tomato Rings	Lamb with Prunes	Pasta with Creamy Broccoli Sauce	Cereal Munch

15	Eggplant Chicken Sandwich	Lamb with Zucchini & Couscous	Asparagus Fried Rice	Coconut Mandarin Salad
16	Eggplant Caprese	Pork with Bell Pepper	Tex-Mex Pepper Stir-Fry	Cream dipped Cucumbers
17	Chorizo Bowl with Corn	Chicken Tortillas	Vegetarian Taco Salad	Barbecue Cups
18	Panzanella Salad	Slow-roast Chicken with Homemade Gravy	Creamy Red Pepper Pasta	Spiced Pretzels
19	Shrimp Bruschetta	Balsamic Chicken Mix	Herbed Mushroom Burgers	Cauliflower with Mustard Sauce
20	Strawberry Muesli	Turkey Pinwheels	Chickpea Curry	Pineapple Cabbage Coleslaw
21	Yogurt Bulgur	Salsa Chicken	Veggie Cabbage Stir-Fry	Seafood Croquettes

Chapter 6: Breakfast

BREAKFAST SALAD FROM GRAINS AND FRUITS	FRENCH TOAST WITH APPLESAUCE
Preparation time: 5 minutes Cooking time: 15 minutes Servings: 6 **Ingredients:** 1 8-oz low fat vanilla yogurt 1 cup raisins 1 orange 1 Red delicious apple 1 Granny Smith apple ¾ cup bulgur ¾ cup quick cooking brown rice ¼ teaspoon salt 3 cups water **Direction:** On high fire, place a large pot and bring water to a boil. Add bulgur and rice. Lower fire to a simmer and cooks for ten minutes while covered. Turn off fire, set aside for 2 minutes while covered. In baking sheet, transfer and evenly spread grains to cool. Meanwhile, peel oranges and cut into sections. Chop and core apples. Once grains are cool, transfer to a large serving bowl along with fruits. Add yogurt and mix well to coat. Serve and enjoy. **Nutrition:** Calories: 187 | Carbs: g; | Protein: g; | Fats: g; | Phosphorus: mg; | Potassium: mg; | Sodium: 117mg	*Preparation time: 5 minutes* *Cooking time: 15 minutes* *Servings: 6* **Ingredients:** *¼ cup unsweetened applesauce* *½ cup milk* *1 teaspoon ground cinnamon* *2 eggs* *2 tablespoon white sugar* *6 slices whole wheat bread* **Directions:** Mix well applesauce, sugar, cinnamon, milk and eggs in a mixing bowl. Dip the bread into applesauce mixture until wet, take note that you should do this one slice at a time. On medium fire, heat a nonstick skillet greased with cooking spray. Add soaked bread one at a time and cook for 2-3 minutes per side or until lightly browned. Serve and enjoy. **Nutrition:** *Calories: 57 |Carbs: 6g | Protein: 4g | Fats: 4g | Phosphorus: 69mg | Potassium: 88mg | Sodium: 43mg*

BAGELS MADE HEALTHY

Preparation time: 5 minutes
Cooking time: 25 minutes
Servings: 8
Ingredients:
2 teaspoon yeast
1 ½ tablespoon olive oil
1 ¼ cups bread flour
2 cups whole wheat flour
1 tablespoon vinegar
2 tablespoon honey
1 ½ cups warm water
Directions:
In a bread machine, mix all ingredients, and then process on dough cycle.
Once done or end of cycle, create 8 pieces shaped like a flattened ball.
Using your thumb, you must create a hole at the center of each then create a donut shape.
In a greased baking sheet, place donut-shaped dough then covers and let it rise about ½ hour.
Prepare about 2 inches of water to boil in a large pan.
In a boiling water, drop one at a time the bagels and boil for 1 minute, then turn them once.
Remove them and return them to baking sheet and bake at 350oF (175oC) for about 20 to 25 minutes until golden brown.
Nutrition:
Calories: 221 | Carbs: 42g | Protein: 7g | Fats: g | Phosphorus: 130mg | Potassium: 166mg | Sodium: 47mg

CORNBREAD WITH SOUTHERN TWIST

Preparation time: 15 minutes
Cooking time: 60 minutes
Servings: 8
Ingredients:
2 tablespoons shortening
1 ¼ cups skim milk
¼ cup egg substitute
4 tablespoons sodium free baking powder
½ cup flour
1 ½ cups cornmeal
Directions:
Prepare 8 x 8-inch baking dish or a black iron skillet then add shortening.
Put the baking dish or skillet inside the oven on 425oF, once the shortening has melted that means the pan is hot already.
In a bowl, add milk and egg then mix well.
Take out the skillet and add the melted shortening into the batter and stir well.
Pour mixture into skillet after mixing all ingredients.
Cook the cornbread for 15-20 minutes until it is golden brown.
Nutrition:
Calories: 166 |Carbs: 35g | Protein: 5g | Fats: 1g | Phosphorus: 79mg | Potassium: 122mg | Sodium: 34mg

GRANDMA'S PANCAKE SPECIAL	VERY BERRY SMOOTHIE
Preparation time: 5 minutes *Cooking time: 15 minutes* *Servings: 3* **Ingredients:** *1 tablespoon oil* *1 cup milk* *1 egg* *2 teaspoons sodium free baking powder* *2 tablespoons sugar* *1 ¼ cups flour* **Directions:** Mix together all the dry ingredients such as the flour, sugar and baking powder. Combine oil, milk and egg in another bowl. Once done, add them all to the flour mixture. Make sure that as your stir the mixture, blend them together until slightly lumpy. In a hot greased griddle, pour-in at least ¼ cup of the batter to make each pancake. To cook, ensure that the bottom is a bit brown, then turn and cook the other side, as well. **Nutrition:** *Calories: 167 | Carbs: 50g | Protein: 11g | Fats: 11g | Phosphorus: 176mg | Potassium: 215mg | Sodium: 70mg*	*Preparation time: 3 minutes* *Cooking time: 5 minutes* *Servings: 2* **Ingredients:** *2 quarts water* *2 cups pomegranate seeds* *1 cup blackberries* *1 cup blueberries* **Directions:** Mix all ingredients in a blender. Puree until smooth and creamy. Transfer to a serving glass and enjoy. **Nutrition:** *Calories: 464 | Carbs: 111g | Protein: 8g | Fats: 4g | Phosphorus: 132mg | Potassium: 843mg | Sodium: 16mg*

PASTA WITH INDIAN LENTILS	APPLE PUMPKIN MUFFINS
Preparation time: 5 minutes *Cooking time: 0 minutes* *Servings: 6* **Ingredients:** *¼-½ cup fresh cilantro (chopped)* *3 cups water* *2 small dry red peppers (whole)* *1 teaspoon turmeric* *1 teaspoon ground cumin* *2-3 cloves garlic (minced)* *1 can diced tomatoes (w/juice)* *1 large onion (chopped)* *½ cup dry lentils (rinsed)* *½ cup orzo or tiny pasta* **Directions:** Combine all ingredients in the skillet except for the cilantro then boil on medium-high heat. Ensure to cover and slightly reduce heat to medium-low and simmer until pasta is tender for about 35 minutes. Afterwards, take out the chili peppers then add cilantro and top it with low-fat sour cream. **Nutrition:** *Calories: 175	Carbs: 40g	Protein: 3g	Fats: 2g	Phosphorus: 139mg	Potassium: 513mg	Sodium: 61mg*	*Preparation Time: 15 minutes* *Cooking Time: 20 minutes* *Servings: 12* **Ingredients** *1 cup all-purpose flour* *1 cup wheat bran* *2 teaspoons phosphorus powder* *1 cup pumpkin purée* *¼ cup honey* *¼ cup olive oil* *1 egg* *1 teaspoon vanilla extract* *½ cup cored diced apple* **Directions** Preheat the oven to 400°f. Line 12 muffin cups with paper liners. Stir together the flour, wheat bran, and baking powder, mix this in a medium bowl. In a small bowl, whisk together the pumpkin, honey, olive oil, egg, and vanilla. Stir the pumpkin mixture into the flour mixture until just combined. Stir in the diced apple. Spoon the batter in the muffin cups. Bake for about 20 minutes, or until a toothpick inserted in the center of a muffin comes out clean. **Nutrition:** *Calories: 125	Total fat: 5g	Saturated fat: 1g	Cholesterol: 18mg	Sodium: 8mg |Carbohydrates: 20g |Fiber: 3g |Phosphorus: 120mg	Potassium: 177mg	Protein: 2g*

SPICED FRENCH TOAST	BREAKFAST TACOS
Preparation time: 15 minutes *Cooking time: 12 minutes* *Servings: 4* **Ingredients** *4 eggs* *½ cup homemade rice milk (here, or use* *unsweetened store-bought) or almond milk* *¼ cup freshly squeezed orange juice* *1 teaspoon ground cinnamon* *½ teaspoon ground ginger* *Pinch ground cloves* *1 tablespoon unsalted butter, divided* *8 slices white bread* **Directions** Whisk eggs, rice milk, orange juice, cinnamon, ginger, and cloves until well blended in a large bowl. Melt half the butter in a large skillet. It should be in medium-high heat only. Dredge four of the bread slices in the egg mixture until well soaked, and place them in the skillet. Cook the toast until golden brown on both sides, turning once, about 6 minutes total. Repeat with the remaining butter and bread. Serve 2 pieces of hot french toast to each person. **Nutrition** *Calories: 236	Total fat: 11g	Saturated fat: 4g |* *Cholesterol: 220mg	Sodium: 84mg |* *Carbohydrates: 27g	Fiber: 1g| Phosphorus:* *119mg	Potassium: 158mg	Protein: 11g*	*Preparation time: 10 minutes* *Cooking time: 10 minutes* *Servings: 4* **Ingredients** *1 teaspoon olive oil* *½ sweet onion, chopped* *½ red bell pepper, chopped* *½ teaspoon minced garlic* *4 eggs, beaten* *½ teaspoon ground cumin* *Pinch red pepper flakes* *4 tortillas* *¼ cup tomato salsa* **Directions** Heat the oil in a large skillet in a medium heat only. Add the onion, bell pepper, and garlic, and sauté until softened, about 5 minutes. Add the eggs, cumin, and red pepper flakes, and scramble the eggs with the vegetables until cooked through and fluffy. Spoon one-fourth of the egg mixture into the center of each tortilla, and top each with 1 tablespoon of salsa. Serve immediately. **Nutrition per serving:** *Calories: 211	Total fat: 7g	Saturated fat: 2g |* *Cholesterol: 211mg	Sodium: 346mg |* *Carbohydrates: 17g	Fiber: 1g	Phosphorus:* *120mg |Potassium: 141mg	Protein: 9g*

MEXICAN SCRAMBLED EGGS IN TORTILLA	AMERICAN BLUEBERRY PANCAKES
Preparation time: 5 minutes *Cooking time: 2 minutes* *Servings: 2* **Ingredients** *2 medium corn tortillas* *4 egg whites* *1 teaspoon of cumin* *3 teaspoons of green chilies, diced* *½ teaspoon of hot pepper sauce* *2 tablespoons of salsa* *½ teaspoon salt* **Directions** Spray some cooking spray on a medium skillet and heat for a few seconds. Whisk the eggs with the green chilies, hot sauce, and comminute Add the eggs into the pan, and whisk with a spatula to scramble. Add the salt. Cook until fluffy and done (1-2 minutes) over low heat. Open the tortillas and spread 1 tablespoon of salsa on each. Distribute the egg mixture onto the tortillas and wrap gently to make a burrito. Serve warm. **Nutrition:** *Calories: 44.1 kcal | Carbohydrate: 2.23 g | Protein: 7.69 g | Sodium: 854 mg | Potassium: 189 mg | Phosphorus: 22 mg | Dietary fiber: 0.5 g | Fat: 0.39 g*	*Preparation time: 5 minutes* *Cooking time: 10 minutes* *Servings: 6* **Ingredients** *1 ½ cups of all-purpose flour, sifted* *1 cup of buttermilk* *3 tablespoons of sugar* *2 tablespoons of unsalted butter, melted* *2 teaspoon of baking powder* *2 eggs, beaten* *1 cup of canned blueberries, rinsed* **Directions** Combine the baking powder, flour and sugar in a bowl. Make a hole in the center and slowly add the rest of the ingredients. Begin to stir gently from the sides to the center with a spatula, until you get a smooth and creamy batter. With cooking spray, spray the pan and place over medium heat. Take one measuring cup and fill 1/3rd of its capacity with the batter to make each pancake. Use a spoon to pour the pancake batter and let cook until golden brown. Flip once to cook the other side. Serve warm with optional agave syrup. **Nutrition:** *Calories: 251.69 kcal | Carbohydrate: 41.68 g |Protein: 7.2 g | Sodium: 186.68 mg | Potassium: 142.87 mg | Phosphorus: 255.39 mg | Dietary fiber: 1.9 g | Fat: 6.47 g*

RASPBERRY PEACH BREAKFAST SMOOTHIE	FAST MICROWAVE EGG SCRAMBLE
Preparation time: 5 minutes *Cooking time: 1 minute* *Servings: 2* **Ingredients** *1/3 cup of raspberries, (it can be frozen)* *1/2 peach, skin and pit removed* *1 tablespoon of honey* *1 cup of coconut water* **Directions** Mix all ingredients together and blend it until smooth. Pour and serve chilled in a tall glass or mason jar. **Nutrition:** *Calories: 86.3 kcal	Carbohydrate: 20.6 g	Protein: 1.4 g	Sodium: 3 mg	Potassium: 109 mg	Phosphorus: 36.08 mg	Dietary fiber: 2.6 g	Fat: 0.31 g*	*Preparation time: 5 minutes* *Cooking time: 1-2 minutes* *Servings: 1* **Ingredients** *1 large egg* *2 large egg whites* *2 tablespoons of milk* *Kosher pepper, ground* **Directions** Spray a coffee cup with a bit of cooking spray. Whisk all the ingredients together and place into the coffee cup. Place the cup with the eggs into the microwave and set to cook for approx. 45 seconds. Take out and stir. Cook it for another 30 seconds after returning it to the microwave. Serve. **Nutrition:** Calories: 128.6 kcal	Carbohydrate: 2.47 g	Protein: 12.96 g	Sodium: 286.36 mg	Potassium: 185.28 mg	Phosphorus: 122.22 mg	Dietary fiber: 0 g	Fat: 5.96 g

MANGO LASSI SMOOTHIE

Preparation time: 5 minutes
Cooking time: 0 minute
Servings: 2
Ingredients
½ cup of plain yogurt
½ cup of plain water
½ cup of sliced mango
1 tablespoon of sugar
¼ teaspoon of cardamom
¼ teaspoon cinnamon
¼ cup lime juice
Directions
Pulse all the above ingredients in a blender until smooth (around 1 minute).
Pour into tall glasses or mason jars and serve chilled immediately.
Nutrition:
Calories: 89.02 kcal | Carbohydrate: 14.31 g | Protein: 2.54 g | Sodium: 30 mg | Potassium: 185.67 mg | Phosphorus: 67.88 mg | Dietary fiber: 0.77 g | Fat: 2.05 g

BREAKFAST MAPLE SAUSAGE

Preparation time: 15 minutes
Cooking time: 8 minutes
Servings: 12
Ingredients
1 pound of pork, minced
½ pound lean turkey meat, ground
¼ teaspoon of nutmeg
½ teaspoon black pepper
¼ all spice
2 tablespoon of maple syrup
1 tablespoon of water
Directions
Combine all the ingredients in a bowl.
Cover and refrigerate for 3-4 hours.
Take the mixture and form into small flat patties with your hand (around 10-12 patties).
Lightly grease a medium skillet with oil and shallow fry the patties over medium to high heat, until brown (around 4-5 minutes on each side).
Serve hot.

Nutrition:
Calories: 53.85 kcal | Carbohydrate: 2.42 g | Protein: 8.5 g | Sodium: 30.96 mg | Potassium: 84.68 mg | Phosphorus: 83.49 mg | Dietary fiber: 0.03 g | Fat: 0.9 g

SUMMER VEGGIE OMELET

Preparation time: 5 minutes
Cooking time: 5 minutes
Servings: 2

Ingredients

4 large egg whites
¼ cup of sweet corn, frozen
⅓ cup of zucchini, grated
2 green onions, sliced
1 tablespoon of cream cheese
Kosher pepper

Directions

Grease a medium pan with some cooking spray and add the onions, corn and grated zucchini.

Sauté for a couple of minutes until softened.

Beat the eggs together with the water, cream cheese, and pepper in a bowl.

Add the eggs into the veggie mixture in the pan, and let cook while moving the edges from inside to outside with a spatula, to allow raw egg to cook through the edges.

Turn the omelet with the aid of a dish (placed over the pan and flipped upside down and then back to the pan).

Let sit for another 1-2 minutes.

Fold in half and serve.

Nutrition:

Calories: 90 kcal | Carbohydrate: 15.97 g | Protein: 8.07 g | Sodium: 227 mg | Potassium: 244.24 mg | Phosphorus: 45.32 mg | Dietary fiber: 0.88 g | Fat: 2.44 g

CHAPTER 7: Breakfast 2

RASPBERRY OVERNIGHT PORRIDGE

Preparation time: overnight
Cooking time: 0 minute
Servings:12
Ingredients
⅓ cup of rolled oats
½ cup almond milk
1 tablespoon of honey
5-6 raspberries, fresh or canned and unsweetened
⅓ cup of rolled oats
½ cup almond milk
1 tablespoon of honey
5-6 raspberries, fresh or canned and unsweetened
Directions
Combine the oats, almond milk, and honey in a mason jar and place into the fridge for overnight. Serve the next morning with the raspberries on top.
Nutrition:
Calories: 143.6 kcal | Carbohydrate: 34.62 g | Protein: 3.44 g | Sodium: 77.88 mg | Potassium: 153.25 mg | Phosphorus: 99.3 mg | Dietary fiber: 7.56 g | Fat: 3.91 g

CHEESY SCRAMBLED EGGS WITH FRESH HERBS

Preparation time: 15 minutes
Cooking time: 10 minutes
Servings: 4
Ingredients
Eggs – 3
Egg whites – 2
Cream cheese – ½ cup
Unsweetened rice milk – ¼ cup
Chopped scallion – 1 tablespoon green part only
Chopped fresh tarragon – 1 tablespoon
Unsalted butter – 2 tablespoons.
Ground black pepper to taste
Directions
In a container, mix the eggs, egg whites, cream cheese, rice milk, scallions, and tarragon until mixed and smooth.
Melt the butter in a skillet.
Pour in the egg mix and cook, stirring, for 5 minutes or until the eggs are thick and curds creamy.
Season with pepper and serve.

Nutrition:
Calories: 221 | Fat: 19g | Carb: 3g | Phosphorus: 119mg | Potassium: 140mg | Sodium: 193mg| Protein: 8g

TURKEY AND SPINACH SCRAMBLE ON MELBA TOAST	VEGETABLE OMELET
Preparation time: 2 minutes *Cooking time: 15 minutes* *Servings: 2* **Ingredients** *Extra virgin olive oil – 1 teaspoon* *Raw spinach – 1 cup* *Garlic – ½ clove, minced* *Nutmeg – 1 teaspoon grated* *Cooked and diced turkey breast – 1 cup* *Melba toast – 4 slices* *Balsamic vinegar – 1 teaspoon* **Directions** Heat a pot over a source of heat and add oil. Add turkey and heat through for 6 to 8 minutes. Add spinach, garlic, and nutmeg and stir-fry for 6 minutes more. Plate up the melba toast and top with spinach and turkey scramble. Drizzle with balsamic vinegar and serve. **Nutrition:** *Calories: 301 | Fat: 19g | Carb: 12g | Phosphorus: 215mg | Potassium: 269mg | Sodium: 360mg | Protein: 19g*	*Preparation time: 15 minutes* *Cooking time: 10 minutes* *Servings: 3* **Ingredients** *Egg whites – 4* *Egg – 1* *Chopped fresh parsley – 2 tablespoons.* *Water – 2 tablespoons.* *Olive oil spray* *Chopped and boiled red bell pepper – ½ cup* *Chopped scallion – ¼ cup, both green and white parts* *Ground black pepper* **Directions** Whisk together the egg, egg whites, parsley, and water until well blended. Set aside. Spray a skillet with olive oil spray and place over medium heat. Sauté the peppers and scallion for 3 minutes or until softened. Over the vegetables, you can now pour the egg and cook, swirling the skillet, for 2 minutes or until the edges start to set. Cook until set. Season with black pepper and serve. **Nutrition:** *Calories: 77 | Fat: 3g | Carb: 2g | Phosphorus: 67mg | Potassium: 194mg | Sodium: 229mg | Protein: 12g*

MEXICAN STYLE BURRITOS	**SWEET PANCAKES**
Preparation time: 5 minutes *Cooking time: 15 minutes* *Servings: 2* **Ingredients** *Olive oil – 1 tablespoon* *Corn tortillas – 2* *Red onion – ¼ cup, chopped* *Red bell peppers – ¼ cup, chopped* *Red chili – ½, deseeded and chopped* *Eggs – 2* *Juice of 1 lime* *Cilantro – 1 tablespoon chopped* **Directions** Turn the broiler to medium heat and place the tortillas underneath for 1 to 2 minutes on each side or until lightly toasted. Remove and keep the broiler on. Sauté onion, chili and bell peppers for 5 to 6 minutes or until soft. Place the eggs on top of the onions and peppers and place skillet under the broiler for 5-6 minutes or until the eggs are cooked. Serve half the eggs and vegetables on top of each tortilla and sprinkle with cilantro and lime juice to serve. **Nutrition:** *Calories: 202 | Fat: 13g | Carb: 19g | Phosphorus: 184mg | Potassium: 233mg | Sodium: 77mg | Protein: 9g*	*Preparation time: 10 minutes* *Cooking time: 5 minutes* *Servings: 5* **Ingredients** *All-purpose flour – 1 cup* *Granulated sugar – 1 tablespoon* *Baking powder – 2 teaspoons.* *Egg whites – 2* *Almond milk - 1 cup* *Olive oil - 2 tablespoons.* *Maple extract – 1 tablespoon* **Directions** Combine the flour, sugar and baking powder in a bowl. Make a well in the center and place to one side. Mx the egg whites, milk, oil, and maple extract, do this in another bowl. Add the egg mixture to the well and gently mix until a batter is formed. Heat skillet over medium heat. Cook 2 minutes on each side or until the pancake is golden only add 1/5 of the batter to the pan. Repeat with the remaining batter and serve. **Nutrition:** *Calories: 178 | Fat potassium: 126mg | Sodium: 297mg | Protein: 6g*

BREAKFAST SMOOTHIE	BUCKWHEAT AND GRAPEFRUIT PORRIDGE
Preparation time: 15 minutes *Cooking time: 0 minute* *Servings: 2* **Ingredients** *Frozen blueberries – 1 cup* *Pineapple chunks – ½ cup* *English cucumber – ½ cup* *Apple – ½* *Water – ½ cup* **Directions** Put the pineapple, blueberries, cucumber, apple, and water in a blender and blend until thick and smooth. Pour into 2 glasses and serve. **Nutrition:** *Calories: 87	Fat: g	Carb: 22g	Phosphorus: 28mg	Potassium: 192mg| Sodium: 3mg| Protein: 0.7g*	*Preparation time: 5 minutes* *Cooking time: 20 minutes* *Servings: 2* **Ingredients** *Buckwheat – ½ cup* *Grapefruit – ¼, chopped* *Honey – 1 tablespoon* *Almond milk – 1 ½ cups* *Water – 2 cups* **Directions** Boil water on the stove. Add the buckwheat and place the lid on the pan. Simmer for 7 to 10 minutes, in a lowheat. Check to ensure water does not dry out. Remove and set aside for 5 minutes, do this when most of the water is absorbed. Drain excess water from the pan and stir in almond milk, heating through for 5 minutes. Add the honey and grapefruit. Serve. **Nutrition:** *Calories: 231	Fat: 4g| Carb: 43g	Phosphorus: 165mg	Potassium: 370mg	Sodium: 135mg*

EGG AND VEGGIE MUFFINS

Preparation time: 15 minutes
Cooking time: 20 minutes
Servings: 4
Ingredients
Cooking spray
Eggs – 4
Unsweetened rice milk – 2 tablespoon
Sweet onion – ½, chopped
Red bell pepper – ½, chopped
Pinch red pepper flakes
Pinch ground black pepper
Directions
Preheat the oven to 350f.
Spray 4 muffin pans with cooking spray. Set aside.
Whisk together the milk, eggs, onion, red pepper, parsley, red pepper flakes, and black pepper until mixed.
Pour the egg mixture into prepared muffin pans.
Bake until the muffins are puffed and golden, about 18 to 20 minutes.
Serve
Nutrition:
Calories: 84 | Fat: 5g | Carb: 3g | Phosphorus: 110mg | Potassium: 117mg | Sodium: 75mg | Protein: 7g

CHERRY BERRY BULGUR BOWL

Preparation time: 15 minutes
Cooking time: 15 minutes
Servings: 4
Ingredients
1 cup medium-grind bulgur
2 cups water
Pinch salt
1 cup halved and pitted cherries or 1 cup canned cherries, drained
½ cup raspberries
½ cup blackberries
1 tablespoon cherry jam
2 cups plain whole-milk yogurt
Directions
Mix the bulgur, water, and salt in a medium saucepan. Do this in a medium heat. Bring to a boil. Reduce the heat to low and simmer, partially covered, for 12 to 15 minutes or until the bulgur is almost tender. Cover, and let stand for 5 minutes to finish cooking do this after removing the pan from the heat.
While the bulgur is cooking, combine the raspberries and blackberries in a medium bowl. Stir the cherry jam into the fruit.
When the bulgur is tender, divide among four bowls. Top each bowl with ½ cup of yogurt and an equal amount of the berry mixture and serve.
Nutrition:
Calories: 242 | Total fat: 6g | Saturated fat: 3g | Sodium: 85mg | Phosphorus: 237mg | Potassium: 438mg | Carbohydrates: 44g | Fiber: 7g | Protein: 9g | Sugar: 13g

BAKED CURRIED APPLE OATMEAL CUPS	MOZZARELLA CHEESE OMELETTE
Preparation time: 10 minutes *Cooking time: 20 minutes* *Servings: 6* **Ingredients** *3½ cups old-fashioned oats* *3 tablespoons brown sugar* *2 teaspoons of your preferred curry powder* *⅛ teaspoon salt* *1 cup unsweetened almond milk* *1 cup unsweetened applesauce* *1 teaspoon vanilla* *½ cup chopped walnuts* **Directions** Preheat the oven to 375°f. Then spray a 12-cup muffin tin with baking spray then set aside. Combine the oats, brown sugar, curry powder, and salt, and mix in a medium bowl. Mix together the milk, applesauce, and vanilla in a small bowl, Stir the liquid ingredients into the dry ingredients and mix until just combined. Stir in the walnuts. Using a scant ⅓ cup for each divide the mixture among the muffin cups. Bake this for 18 to 20 minutes until the oatmeal is firm. Serve. **Nutrition:** *For 2 oatmeal cups: Calories: 296 | Total fat: 10g | Saturated fat: 1g | Sodium: 84mg | Phosphorus: 236mg | Potassium: 289mg | Carbohydrates: 45g | Fiber: 6g | Protein: 8g | Sugar: 11g*	*Preparation time: 10 minutes* *Cooking time: 5 minutes* *Servings: 1* **Ingredients:** *4 eggs, beaten* *1/4 cup mozzarella cheese, shredded* *4 tomato slices* *1/4 tsp italian seasoning* *1/4 tsp dried oregano* *Pepper* *Salt* **Directions:** In a small bowl, whisk eggs with salt. Spray pan with cooking spray and heat over medium heat. Pour egg mixture into the pan and cook over medium heat. Once eggs are set then sprinkle oregano and italian seasoning on top. Arrange tomato slices on top of the omelet and sprinkle with shredded cheese. Cook omelet for 1 minute. Serve and enjoy. **Nutrition:** *Calories 285 | Fat 19 g | Carbohydrates 4 g | Sugar 3 g | Protein 25 g | Cholesterol 655 mg*

SUN-DRIED TOMATO FRITTATA	**ITALIAN BREAKFAST FRITTATA**
Preparation time: 10 minutes *Cooking time: 20 minutes* *Servings: 8* **Ingredients:** *12 eggs* *1/2 tsp dried basil* *1/4 cup parmesan cheese, grated* *2 cups baby spinach, shredded* *1/4 cup sun-dried tomatoes, sliced* *Pepper* *Salt* **Directions:** Preheat the oven to 425 f. In a large bowl, whisk eggs with pepper and salt. Add remaining ingredients and stir to combine. Spray oven-safe pan with cooking spray. Pour egg mixture into the pan and bake for 20 minutes. Slice and serve. **Nutrition:** *Calories 115	Fat 7 g	Carbohydrates 1 g	Sugar 1 g	Protein 10 g	Cholesterol 250 mg*	*Preparation time: 10 minutes* *Cooking time: 45 minutes* *Servings: 4* **Ingredients:** *2 cups egg whites* *1/2 cup mozzarella cheese, shredded* *1 cup cottage cheese, crumbled* *1/4 cup fresh basil, sliced* *1/2 cup roasted red peppers, sliced* *Pepper* *Salt* **Directions:** Preheat the oven to 375 f. Add all ingredients into the large bowl and whisk well to combine. Pour frittata mixture into the baking dish and bake for 45 minutes. Slice and serve. **Nutrition:** *Calories 131	Fat 2 g	Carbohydrates 5 g	Sugar 2 g	Protein 22 g	Cholesterol 6 mg*

SAUSAGE CHEESE BAKE OMELETTE	GREEK EGG SCRAMBLED
Preparation time: 10 minutes *Cooking time: 45 minutes* *Servings: 8* **Ingredients:** *16 eggs* *2 cups cheddar cheese, shredded* *1/2 cup salsa* *1 lb ground sausage* *1 1/2 cups coconut milk* *Pepper* *Salt* **Directions:** Preheat the oven to 350 f. Add sausage in a pan and cook until browned. Drain excess fat. In a large bowl, whisk eggs and milk. Stir in cheese, cooked sausage, and salsa. Pour omelet mixture into the baking dish and bake for 45 minutes. Serve and enjoy. **Nutrition:** *Calories 360	Fat 24 g	Carbohydrates 4 g	Sugar 3 g	Protein 28 g	Cholesterol 400 mg*	*Preparation time: 10 minutes* *Cooking time: 10 minutes* *Servings: 2* **Ingredients:** *4 eggs* *1/2 cup grape tomatoes, sliced* *2 tbsp green onions, sliced* *1 bell pepper, diced* *1 tbsp olive oil* *1/4 tsp dried oregano* *1/2 tbsp capers* *3 olives, sliced* *Pepper* *Salt* **Directions:** Heat oil in a pan over medium heat. Add green onions and bell pepper and cook until pepper is softened. Add tomatoes, capers, and olives and cook for 1 minute. Add eggs and stir until eggs are cooked. Season with oregano, pepper, and salt. Serve and enjoy. **Nutrition:** *Calories 230	Fat 17 g	Carbohydrates 8 g	Sugar 5 g	Protein 12 g	Cholesterol 325 mg*

FETA MINT OMELETTE	SAUSAGE CASSEROLE
Preparation time: 10 minutes *Cooking time: 5 minutes* *Servings: 1* **Ingredients:** *3 eggs* *1/4 cup fresh mint, chopped* *2 tbsp coconut milk* *1/2 tsp olive oil* *2 tbsp feta cheese, crumbled* *Pepper* *Salt* **Directions:** In a bowl, whisk eggs with feta cheese, mint, milk, pepper, and salt. Heat olive oil in a pan over low heat. Pour egg mixture in the pan and cook until eggs are set. Flip omelet and cook for 2 minutes more. Serve and enjoy. **Nutrition:** *Calories 275	Fat 20 g	Carbohydrates 4 g	Sugar 2 g	Protein 20 g	Cholesterol 505 mg*	*Preparation time: 10 minutes* *Cooking time: 50 minutes* *Servings: 8* **Ingredients:** *12 eggs* *1 lb. Ground italian sausage* *2 1/2 tomatoes, sliced* *3 tbsp coconut flour* *1/4 cup coconut milk* *2 small zucchinis, shredded* *Pepper* *Salt* **Directions:** Preheat the oven to 350 f. Cook sausage in a pan until brown. Transfer sausage to a mixing bowl. Add coconut flour, milk, eggs, zucchini, pepper, and salt. Stir well. Add eggs and whisk to combine. Transfer bowl mixture into the casserole dish and top with tomato slices. Bake for 50 minutes. Serve and enjoy. **Nutrition:** *Calories 305	Fat 21.8 g	Carbohydrates 6.3 g	Sugar 3.3 g	Protein 19.6 g	Cholesterol 286 mg*

PEANUT BUTTER BREAD PUDDING CUPS

Preparation time: 10 minutes
Cooking time: 20 minutes
Servings: 6
Ingredients
Baking spray
5 slices whole-wheat bread, coarsely crumbled
2 large eggs
½ cup unsweetened almond milk
¼ cup peanut butter
2 tablespoons honey
1 teaspoon vanilla
½ cup chopped unsalted peanuts
Directions
Preheat the oven to 375°f. And then spray a 6-cup muffin tin with baking spray and set aside.
Put the breadcrumbs in a medium bowl.
Beat the eggs, milk, peanut butter, honey, and vanilla until smooth. Pour over the breadcrumbs.
Stir gently until combined, then divide the mixture evenly among the muffin cups. Sprinkle with the peanuts.
Bake this for 18-20 minutes or until the puddings are set. Serve warm.
Nutrition:
For cup: Calories: 261 | Total fat: 15g | Saturated fat: 3g| Sodium: 220mg | Phosphorus: 176mg | Potassium: 261mg | Carbohydrates: 24g | Fiber: 3g | Protein: 12g | Sugar: 9g

DELIGHTFUL PIZZA	WINNER KABOBS
Preparation Time: 40 minutes *Cooking Time: 15 minutes* *Serving: 4* **Ingredients**: *2 (6½-inch) pita breads* *3 tbsp. of low-sodium tomato sauce* *3-ounce of cubed unsalted cooked chicken* *¼ cup of chopped onion* *2 tbsp. of crumbled feta cheese* **Directions**: Preheat the oven to 350 degrees F. Grease a baking sheet. Arrange the pita breads onto prepared baking sheet. Spread the barbecue sauce over each pita bread evenly. Top with chicken and onion evenly and sprinkle with cheese. Bake for about 11-13 minutes. Cut each pizza in half and serve. **Nutrition**: *Calories: 133	Fat: 2g	Carbs: 18.2g	Protein: 9.8g	Fiber: 1g	Sodium: 287mg*	*Preparation Time: 50 minutes* *Cooking Time: 15 minutes* *Serving: 4* **Ingredients**: *1 pound of cubed skinless, boneless chicken breast* *1 seeded and cut into 1-inch pieces medium red bell pepper* *1 seeded and cut into 1-inch pieces medium green bell pepper* *20-ounce of cut into 1-inch pieces pineapple* *1 cut into 1-inch pieces red onion* *1/3 cup of low-sodium barbecue sauce* *Freshly ground black pepper, to taste* **Directions**: Preheat the outdoor grill to medium-high heat. Lightly, grease the grill grate. Thread chicken, bell peppers, pineapple and onion onto pre-soaked 6 wooden skewers. Coat all the ingredients with ½ of barbecue sauce and sprinkle with black pepper. Place the skewers in prepared baking sheet in a single layer. Grill the skewers for about 9-10 minutes, flipping occasionally. Remove from grill and immediately, coat with remaining barbecue sauce. Serve immediately. **Nutrition**: *Calories: 182	Fat: 3g	Carbs: 22.2g	Protein: 18g	Fiber: 2.3g	Potassium: 234mg	Sodium: 185mg*

TEMPTING BURGERS	DOLMAS WRAP
Preparation Time: 20 minutes *Cooking Time: 15 minutes* *Servings: 6* **Ingredients**: *12-ounce of finely chopped unsalted cooked salmon* *½ cup of minced onion* *1 minced garlic clove* *2 tbsp. of chopped fresh parsley* *1 large egg* *½ tsp. of paprika* *Freshly ground black pepper, to taste* *2 tbsp. of olive oil* *3 cups torn lettuce* **Directions**: Preheat the oven to 350 degrees F. Line a baking sheet with parchment paper. In a large bowl, add all ingredients except oil and mix until well combined. Make equal sized 12 patties from mixture. Place patties onto prepared baking dish in a single layer. Bake for about 12-15 minutes. Now, in a large skillet, heat oil on high heat. Remove salmon burgers from oven and transfer into skillet. Cook for about 1 minute per side. Divide lettuce in serving plates evenly. Place 2 patties in each plate and serve. **Nutrition**: *Calories 136	Fat 9.1g	Carbs 2.1g	Protein 12.4g	Fiber 0.5g	Potassium 295mg	Sodium: 39mg*	*Preparation Time: 10 minutes* *Cooking Time: 5 minutes* *Servings: 2* **Ingredients:** *2 whole wheat wraps* *6 dolmas (stuffed grape leaves)* *1 tomato, chopped* *1 cucumber, chopped* *2 oz Greek yogurt* *½ teaspoon minced garlic* *¼ cup lettuce, chopped* *2 oz Feta, crumbled* **Directions:** In the mixing bowl combine together chopped tomato, cucumber, Greek yogurt, minced garlic, lettuce, and Feta. When the mixture is homogenous transfer it in the center of every wheat wrap. Arrange dolma over the vegetable mixture. Carefully wrap the wheat wraps. **Nutrition:** *Calories 341	Fat 12.9	Fiber 9.2	Carbs 52.4	Protein 13.2*

SALAD TO TONNO

Preparation Time: 15 minutes
Cooking Time: 0 minutes
Servings: 2
Ingredients:
1/3 cup stuffed green olives
1 ½ cup lettuce leaves
½ cup cherry tomatoes, halved
½ teaspoon garlic powder
½ teaspoon salt
½ teaspoon ground black pepper
1 tablespoon lemon juice
1 teaspoon olive oil
6 oz tuna, canned, drained
Directions:
Chop the tuna roughly and put it in the salad bowl.
Add cherry tomatoes, lettuce leaves, salt, garlic powder, ground black pepper. Lemon juice, and olive oil.
Then slice the stuffed olives and add them in the salad too.
Give a good shake to the salad.
Salad can be stored in the fridge for up to 3 hours.
Nutrition:
Calories 235 | Fat 12 | Fiber 1 | Carbs 6.5 | Protein 23.4

ARLECCHINO RICE SALAD

Preparation Time: 10 minutes
Cooking Time: 15 minutes
Servings: 3
Ingredients:
½ cup white rice, dried
1 cup chicken stock
1 zucchini, shredded
2 tablespoons capers
1 carrot, shredded
1 tomato, chopped
1 tablespoon apple cider vinegar
½ teaspoon salt
2 tablespoons fresh parsley, chopped
1 tablespoon canola oil
Directions:
Put rice in the pan.
Add chicken stock and boil it with the closed lid for 15-20 minutes or until rice absorbs all water.
Meanwhile, in the mixing bowl combine together shredded zucchini, capers, carrot, and tomato.
Add fresh parsley.
Make the dressing: mix up together canola oil, salt, and apple cider vinegar.
Chill the cooked rice little and add it in the salad bowl to the vegetables.
Add dressing and mix up salad well.
Nutrition:
Calories 183 | Fat 5.3 | Fiber 2.1 | Carbs 30.4 | Protein 3.8

GREEK SALAD	SAUTÉED CHICKPEA AND LENTIL MIX
Preparation Time: 10 minutes *Cooking Time: 0 minutes* *Servings: 2* **Ingredients:** *2 cups lettuce leaves* *4 oz black olives* *2 tomatoes* *2 cucumbers* *1 tablespoon lemon juice* *1 teaspoon olive oil* *¼ teaspoon dried oregano* *½ teaspoon salt* *¼ teaspoon chili flakes* *4 oz Feta cheese* **Directions:** Chop Feta cheese into the small cubes. Chop the lettuce leaves roughly put them in the salad bowl. Slice black olives and add them in the lettuce. Then chop tomatoes and cucumbers into the cubes. Add them in the lettuce bowl. For the dressing: whisk together chili flakes, salt, dried oregano, olive oil, and lemon juice. Pour the dressing over the lettuce mixture and mix up well. Sprinkle the salad with Feta cubes and shake gently. **Nutrition:** *Calories 312	Fat 21.2	Fiber 5.3	Carbs 23.5	Protein 11.9*	*Preparation Time: 10 minutes* *Cooking Time: 50 minutes* *Servings: 4* **Ingredients:** *1 cup chickpeas, half-cooked* *1 cup lentils* *5 cups chicken stock* *½ cup fresh cilantro, chopped* *1 teaspoon salt* *½ teaspoon chili flakes* *¼ cup onion, diced* *1 tablespoon tomato paste* **Directions:** Place chickpeas in the pan. Add water, salt, and chili flakes. Boil the chickpeas for 30 minutes over the medium heat. Then add diced onion, lentils, and tomato paste. Stir well. Close the lid and cook the mix for 15 minutes. After this, add chopped cilantro, stir the meal well and cook it for 5 minutes more. Let the cooked lunch chill little before serving. **Nutrition:** *Calories 370	Fat 4.3	Fiber 23.7	Carbs 61.6	Protein 23.2*

BUFFALO CHICKEN LETTUCE WRAPS

Preparation Time: 35 minutes
Cooking Time: 10 minutes
Servings: 2
Ingredients:
3 chicken breasts, boneless and cubed
20 slices of almond butter lettuce leaves
¾ cup cherry tomatoes halved
1 avocado, chopped
¼ cup green onions, diced
½ cup ranch dressing
¾ cup hot sauce
Directions:
Take a mixing bowl and add chicken cubes and hot sauce, mix.
Place in the fridge and let it marinate for 30 minutes.
Preheat your oven to 400 degrees F.
Place coated chicken on a cookie pan and bake for 9 minutes.
Assemble lettuce serving cups with equal amounts of lettuce, green onions, tomatoes, ranch dressing, and cubed chicken.
Serve and enjoy!
Nutrition:
Calories 106 | Fat 6g | Carbohydrates 2g | Protein 5g

CRAZY JAPANESE POTATO AND BEEF CROQUETTES

Preparation Time: 10 minutes
Cooking Time: 20 minutes
Servings: 10
Ingredients:
3 medium russet potatoes, peeled and chopped
1 tablespoon almond butter
1 tablespoon vegetable oil
3 onions, diced
¾ pound ground beef
4 teaspoons light coconut aminos
All-purpose flour for coating
2 eggs, beaten
Panko bread crumbs for coating
½ cup oil, frying
Directions:
Take a saucepan and place it over medium-high heat; add potatoes and sunflower seeds water, boil for 16 minutes.
Remove water and put potatoes in another bowl, add almond butter and mash the potatoes.
Take a frying pan and place it over medium heat, add 1 tablespoon oil and let it heat up.
Add onions and stir fry until tender.
Add coconut aminos to beef to onions.
Keep frying until beef is browned.
Mix the beef with the potatoes evenly.
Take another frying pan and place it over medium heat; add half a cup of oil.
Form croquettes using the mashed potato mixture and coat them with flour, then eggs and finally breadcrumbs. Fry patties until golden on all sides.
Enjoy!
Nutrition:
Calories 239 | Fat 4g | Carbohydrates 20g | Protein 10g

SPICY CHILI CRACKERS	**GOLDEN EGGPLANT FRIES**
Preparation Time: 15 minutes *Cooking Time: 60 minutes* *Servings: 30 crackers* **Ingredients:** *¾ cup almond flour* *¼ cup coconut four* *¼ cup coconut flour* *½ teaspoon paprika* *½ teaspoon cumin* *1 ½ teaspoons chili pepper spice* *1 teaspoon onion powder* *½ teaspoon sunflower seeds* *1 whole egg* *¼ cup unsalted almond butter* **Directions:** Preheat your oven to 350 degrees F. Line a baking sheet with parchment paper and keep it on the side. Add ingredients to your food processor and pulse until you have a nice dough. Divide dough into two equal parts. Place one ball on a sheet of parchment paper and cover with another sheet; roll it out. Cut into crackers and repeat with the other ball. Transfer the prepped dough to a baking tray and bake for 8-10 minutes. Remove from oven and serve. Enjoy! **Nutrition:** *Carbs: 2.8g | Fiber: 1g | Protein: 1.6g | Fat: 4.1g*	*Preparation Time: 10 minutes* *Cooking Time: 15 minutes* *Servings: 8* **Ingredients:** *2 eggs* *2 cups almond flour* *2 tablespoons coconut oil, spray* *2 eggplant, peeled and cut thinly* *Sunflower seeds and pepper* **Directions:** Preheat your oven to 400 degrees F. Take a bowl and mix with sunflower seeds and black pepper. Take another bowl and beat eggs until frothy. Dip the eggplant pieces into the eggs. Then coat them with the flour mixture. Add another layer of flour and egg. Then, take a baking sheet and grease with coconut oil on top. Bake for about 15 minutes. Serve and enjoy! **Nutrition:** *Calories: 212 | Fat: 15.8g | Carbohydrates: 12.1g | Protein: 8.6g*

TRADITIONAL BLACK BEAN CHILI	VERY WILD MUSHROOM PILAF
Preparation Time: 10 minutes *Cooking Time: 4 hours* *Servings: 4* **Ingredients:** *1 ½ cups red bell pepper, chopped* *1 cup yellow onion, chopped* *1 ½ cups mushrooms, sliced* *1 tablespoon olive oil* *1 tablespoon chili powder* *2 garlic cloves, minced* *1 teaspoon chipotle chili pepper, chopped* *½ teaspoon cumin, ground* *16 ounces canned black beans, drained and rinsed* *2 tablespoons cilantro, chopped* *1 cup tomatoes, chopped* **Directions:** Add red bell peppers, onion, dill, mushrooms, chili powder, garlic, chili pepper, cumin, black beans, and tomatoes to your Slow Cooker. Stir well. Place lid and cook on HIGH for 4 hours. Sprinkle cilantro on top. Serve and enjoy! **Nutrition:** *Calories: 211	Fat: 3g	Carbohydrates: 22g	Protein: 5g*	*Preparation Time: 10 minutes* *Cooking Time: 3 hours* *Servings: 4* **Ingredients:** *1 cup wild rice* *2 garlic cloves, minced* *6 green onions, chopped* *2 tablespoons olive oil* *½ pound baby Bella mushrooms* *2 cups water* **Directions:** Add rice, garlic, onion, oil, mushrooms and water to your Slow Cooker. Stir well until mixed. Place lid and cook on LOW for 3 hours. Stir pilaf and divide between serving platters. Enjoy! **Nutrition:** *Calories: 210	Fat: 7g	Carbohydrates: 16g	Protein: 4g*

GREEN PALAK PANEER

Preparation Time: 5 minutes
Cooking Time: 10 minutes
Servings: 4
Ingredients:
1-pound spinach
2 cups cubed paneer (vegan)
2 tablespoons coconut oil
1 teaspoon cumin
1 chopped up onion
1-2 teaspoons hot green chili minced up
1 teaspoon minced garlic
15 cashews
4 tablespoons almond milk
1 teaspoon Garam masala
Flavored vinegar as needed
Directions:
Add cashews and milk to a blender and blend well.
Set your pot to Sauté mode and add coconut oil; allow the oil to heat up.
Add cumin seeds, garlic, green chilies, ginger and sauté for 1 minute.
Add onion and sauté for 2 minutes.
Add chopped spinach, flavored vinegar and a cup of water.
Lock up the lid and cook on HIGH pressure for 10 minutes.
Quick-release the pressure
Add ½ cup of water and blend to a paste.
Add cashew paste, paneer and Garam Masala and stir thoroughly.
Serve over hot rice!
Nutrition:
Calories 367 | Fat 26g | Carbohydrates 21g | Protein 16g

Chapter 9: Lunch 2

SPORTY BABY CARROTS	SAUCY GARLIC GREENS
Preparation Time: 5 minutes *Cooking Time: 5 minutes* *Servings: 4* **Ingredients:** *1-pound baby carrots* *1 cup water* *1 tablespoon clarified ghee* *1 tablespoon chopped up fresh mint leaves* *Sea flavored vinegar as needed* **Directions:** Place a steamer rack on top of your pot and add the carrots. Add water. Lock the lid and cook at HIGH pressure for 2 minutes. Do a quick release. Pass the carrots through a strainer and drain them. Wipe the insert clean. Return the insert to the pot and set the pot to Sauté mode. Add clarified butter and allow it to melt. Add mint and sauté for 30 seconds. Add carrots to the insert and sauté well. Remove them and sprinkle with bit of flavored vinegar on top. Enjoy! **Nutrition:** *Calories: 131	Fat: 10g	Carbohydrates: 11g	Protein: 1g*	*Preparation Time: 5 minutes* *Cooking Time: 20 minutes* *Servings: 4* **Ingredients:** *1 bunch of leafy greens* *Sauce* *½ cup cashews soaked in water for 10 minutes* *¼ cup water* *1 tablespoon lemon juice* *1 teaspoon coconut aminos* *1 clove peeled whole clove* *1/8 teaspoon of flavored vinegar* **Directions:** Make the sauce by draining and discarding the soaking water from your cashews and add the cashews to a blender. Add fresh water, lemon juice, flavored vinegar, coconut aminos, garlic. Blitz until you have a smooth cream and transfer to bowl. Add ½ cup of water to the pot. Place the steamer basket to the pot and add the greens in the basket. Lock the lid and steam for 1 minute. Quick-release the pressure Transfer the steamed greens to strainer and extract excess water. Place the greens into a mixing bowl. Add lemon garlic sauce and toss. Enjoy! **Nutrition:** *Calories: 77	Fat: 5g	Carbohydrates: 0g	Protein: 2g*

CHICKEN NOODLE SOUP	CARROT CASSEROLE
Preparation Time: 15 minutes *Cooking Time: 25 minutes* *Servings: 4* **Ingredients:** *1 cup low-sodium chicken broth* *1 cup water* *1/4 teaspoon poultry seasoning* *1/4 teaspoon black pepper* *1/4 cup carrot, chopped* *1 cup chicken, cooked and shredded* *2 ounces egg noodles* **Direction:** Add broth and water in a slow cooker. Set the pot to high. Add poultry seasoning and pepper. Add carrot, chicken and egg noodles to the pot. Cook on high setting for 25 minutes. Serve while warm. **Nutrition:** *Calories 141	Protein 15g	Carbohydrates 11g |* *Fat 4g	Sodium 191mg	Potassium 135mg |* *Phosphorus 104mg	Calcium 16mg	Fiber 0.7 g*	*Preparation Time: 10 minutes* *Cooking Time: 20 minutes* *Serving: 8* **Ingredients:** *1 lb. carrots, sliced into rounds* *12 low-sodium crackers* *2 tablespoons butter* *2 tablespoons onion, chopped* *1/4 cup cheddar cheese, shredded* **Direction:** Preheat your oven to 350 degrees F. Boil carrots in a pot of water until tender. Drain the carrots and reserve ¼ cup liquid. Mash carrots. Add all the **Ingredients** into the carrots except cheese. Place the mashed carrots in a casserole dish. Sprinkle cheese on top and bake in the oven for 15 minutes. **Nutrition:** *Calories 37	Protein 1g	Carbohydrates 4g |* *Sodium 33 mg	Potassium 106 mg	Phosphorus 21mg*

CAULIFLOWER RICE

Preparation Time: 10 minutes
Cooking Time: 10 minutes
Servings: 4
Ingredients:
1 head cauliflower, sliced into florets
1 tablespoon butter
Black pepper to taste
1/4 teaspoon garlic powder
1/4 teaspoon herb seasoning blend
Direction:
Put cauliflower florets in a food processor. Pulse until consistency is similar to grain.
In a pan over medium heat, melt the butter and add the spices. Toss cauliflower rice and cook for 10 minutes.
Fluff using a fork before serving.
Nutrition:
Calories 47| Protein 1g | Carbohydrates 4g | Sodium 43mg | Potassium 206mg | Phosphorus 31mg | Calcium 16mg

CHICKEN PINEAPPLE CURRY

Preparation Time: 40 Minutes
Cooking Time: 3 hours 10 minutes
Servings: 6
Ingredients:
1 1/2 lbs. chicken thighs, boneless, skinless
1/2 teaspoon black pepper
1/2 teaspoon garlic powder
2 tablespoons olive oil
20 oz. canned pineapple
2 tablespoons brown Swerve
2 tablespoons soy sauce
1/2 teaspoon Tabasco sauce
2 tablespoons cornstarch
3 tablespoons water

Direction:
Begin by seasoning the chicken thighs with garlic powder and black pepper.
Set a suitable skillet over medium-high heat and add the oil to heat.
Add the boneless chicken to the skillet and cook for 3 minutes per side.
Transfer this seared chicken to a Slow cooker, greased with cooking spray.
Add 1 cup of the pineapple juice, Swerve, 1 cup of pineapple, tabasco sauce, and soy sauce to a slow cooker.
Cover the chicken-pineapple mixture and cook for 3 hours on low heat.
Transfer the chicken to the serving plates.
Mix the cornstarch with water in a small bowl and pour it into the pineapple curry.
Stir and cook this sauce for 2 minutes on high heat until it thickens.
Pour this sauce over the chicken and garnish with green onions. Serve warm.
Nutrition:
Calories 256 | Fat 10.4g | Cholesterol 67mg | Sodium 371mg | Protein 22.8g | Phosphorous 107mg | Potassium 308mg

BAKED PORK CHOPS	LASAGNA ROLLS IN MARINARA SAUCE
Preparation Time: 20 Minutes *Cooking Time: 40minutes* *Servings: 6* **Ingredients:** *1/2 cup flour* *1 large egg* *1/4 cup water* *3/4 cup breadcrumbs* *6 (3 1/2 oz.) pork chops* *2 tablespoons butter, unsalted* *1 teaspoon paprika* **Direction**: Begin by switching the oven to 350 degrees F to preheat. Mix and spread the flour in a shallow plate. Whisk the egg with water in another shallow bowl. Spread the breadcrumbs on a separate plate. Firstly, coat the pork with flour, then dip in the egg mix and then in the crumbs. Grease a baking sheet and place the chops in it. Drizzle the pepper on top and bake for 40 minutes. Serve. **Nutrition:** *Calories 221 | Sodium 135mg | Carbohydrate 11.9g | Protein 24.7g | Phosphorous 299mg | Potassium 391mg*	*Preparation Time: 15 Minutes* *Cooking Time: 30 minutes* *Servings: 9* **Ingredients:** *¼ tsp crushed red pepper* *¼ tsp salt* *½ cup shredded mozzarella cheese* *½ cups parmesan cheese, shredded* *1 14-oz package tofu, cubed* *1 25-oz can of low-sodium marinara sauce* *1 tbsp extra virgin olive oil* *12 whole wheat lasagna noodles* *2 tbsp Kalamata olives, chopped* *3 cloves minced garlic* *3 cups spinach, chopped* **Direction**s: Put enough water on a large pot and cook the lasagna noodles according to package **Direction**. Drain, rinse and set aside until ready to use. In a large skillet, sauté garlic over medium heat for 20 seconds. Add the tofu and spinach and cook until the spinach wilts. Transfer this mixture in a bowl and add parmesan olives, salt, red pepper and 2/3 cup of the marinara sauce. In a pan, spread a cup of marinara sauce on the bottom. To make the rolls, place noodle on a surface and spread ¼ cup of the tofu filling. Roll up and place it on the pan with the marinara sauce. Do this procedure until all lasagna noodles are rolled. Place the pan over high heat and bring to a simmer. Reduce the heat to medium and let it cook for three more minutes. Sprinkle mozzarella cheese and let the cheese melt for two minutes. Serve hot. **Nutrition:** *Calories: 600 | Carbs: 65g | Protein: 36g | Phosphorus: 627mg | Potassium: 914mg | Sodium: 1194mg*

CHICKEN CURRY

Preparation Time: 10 Minutes
Cooking Time: 9 Hours
Servings: 5
Ingredients:
2 to 3 boneless chicken breasts
¼ Cup of chopped green onions
1 can of 4 oz of diced green chilli peppers
2 Teaspoons of minced garlic
1 and 1/2 teaspoons of curry powder
1 Teaspoon of chili Powder
1 Teaspoon of cumin
½ Teaspoon of cinnamon
1 Teaspoon of lime juice
1 and 1/2 cups water
1 can or 7 oz of coconut milk
2 Cups of white cooked rice
Chopped cilantro, for garnish
Direction:
Combine the green onion with the chicken, the green chilli peppers, the garlic, the curry powder, the chilli powder, the cumin, the cinnamon, the lime juice, and the water in the bottom of a 6-qt slow cooker
Cover the slow cooker with a lid and cook your **Ingredients** on Low for about 7 to 9 hours
After the **Cooking Time** ends up; shred the chicken with the help of a fork
Add in the coconut milk and cook on High for about 15 minutes
Top the chicken with cilantro; then serve your dish with rice
Enjoy your lunch!
Nutrition:
Calories: 254 | Fats: 18g | Carbs: 6g | Fiber: 1.6g | Potassium: 370mg | Sodium: 240mg | Phosphorous: 114mg | Protein 17g

STEAK WITH ONION

Preparation Time: 5 Minutes
Cooking Time: 60 Minutes
Servings: 7-8
Ingredients:
¼ Cup of white flour
1/8 Teaspoon of ground black pepper
1 and ½ pounds of round steak of ¾ inch of thickness each
2 Tablespoons of oil
1 Cup of water
1 tablespoon of vinegar
1 Minced garlic clove
1 to 2 bay leaves
¼ teaspoon of crushed dried thyme
3 Sliced medium onions

Directions:
Cut the steak into about 7 to 8 equal **Servings**.
Combine the flour and the pepper; then pound the **Ingredients** all together into the meat.
Heat the oil in a large skillet over a medium high heat and brown the meat on both its sides
Remove the meat from the skillet and set it aside
Combine the water with the vinegar, the garlic, the bay leaf and the thyme in the skillet; then bring the mixture to a boil
Place the meat in the mixture and cover it with onion slices
Cover your **Ingredients** and let simmer for about 55 to 60 minutes
Serve and enjoy your lunch!
Nutrition:
Calories: 286 | Fats: 18g | Carbs: 12g | Fiber: 2.25g | Potassium: 368mg | Sodium: 45mg | Phosphorous: 180mg | Protein 19g

SHRIMP SCAMPI	CHICKEN PAELLA
Preparation Time: 4 Minutes *Cooking Time: 8 Minutes* *Servings: 3* **Ingredients:** *1 Tablespoon of olive oil* *1 Minced garlic clove* *½ Pound of cleaned and peeled shrimp* *¼ Cup of dry white wine* *1 Tablespoon of lemon juice* *½ teaspoon of basil* *1 tablespoon of chopped fresh parsley* *4 Oz of dry linguini* **Direction**s: Heat the oil in a large non-stick skillet; then add the garlic and the shrimp and cook while stirring for about 4 minutes Add the wine, the lemon juice, the basil and the parsley Cook for about 5 minutes longer; then boil the linguini in unsalted water for a few minutes Drain the linguini; then top it with the shrimp Serve and enjoy your lunch! **Nutrition:** *Calories: 340 | Fats: 26g | Carbs: 11.3g | Fiber: 2.1g | Potassium: 189mg | Sodium: 85mg | Phosphorous: 167mg | Protein 15g*	*Preparation Time: 5 Minutes* *Cooking Time: 10 Minutes* *Servings: 8* **Ingredients:** *½ Pound of skinned, boned and cut into pieces, chicken breasts* *1/4 Cup of water* *1 Can of 10-1/2 oz of low-sodium chicken broth* *½ Pound of peeled and cleaned medium-size shrimp* *1/2 Cup of frozen green pepper* *1/3 cup of chopped red bell* *1/3 cup of thinly sliced green onion* *2 Minced garlic cloves* *1/4 Teaspoon of pepper* *1 Dash of ground saffron* *1 Cup of uncooked instant white rice* **Direction:** Combine the first 3 **Ingredients** in medium casserole and cover it with a lid; then microwave it for about 4 minutes Stir in the shrimp and the following 6 **Ingredients**; then cover and microwave the shrimp on a high heat for about 3 and ½ minutes Stir in the rice; then cover and set aside for about 5 minutes Serve and enjoy your paella! **Nutrition:** *Calories: 236 | Fats: 11g | Carbs: 6g | Fiber: 1.2g | Potassium: 178mg | Sodium: 83mg | Phosphorous: 144mg | Protein 28g*

BEEF KABOBS WITH PEPPER

Preparation Time: 5 Minutes
Cooking Time: 10 Minutes
Servings: 8
Ingredients:
1 Pound of beef sirloin
½ Cup of vinegar
2 tbsp of salad oil
1 Medium, chopped onion
2 tbsp of chopped fresh parsley
¼ tsp of black pepper
2 Cut into strips green peppers
Directions*:*
Trim the fat from the meat; then cut it into cubes of 1 and ½ inches each
Mix the vinegar, the oil, the onion, the parsley and the pepper in a bowl
Place the meat in the marinade and set it aside for about 2 hours; make sure to stir from time to time.
Remove the meat from the marinade and alternate it on skewers instead with green pepper
Brush the pepper with the marinade and broil for about 10 minutes 4 inches from the heat
Serve and enjoy your kabobs
Nutrition:
Calories: 357 | Fats: 24g | Carbs: 9g | Fiber: 2.3g | Potassium: 250mg | Sodium: 60mg | Phosphorous: 217mg | Protein 26g

Chapter 10: Smoothies and Drinks

BLUEBERRY BLAST SMOOTHIE	PINEAPPLE PROTEIN SMOOTHIE
Preparation Time: 10minutes *Cooking Time: 0 minutes* *Servings: 1* **Ingredients:** *1 cup frozen blueberries* *8 packets of Splenda* *6 tbsp of protein powder* *8 ice cubes* *14 oz apple juice* **Directions:** First, start by putting all the ingredients in a blender jug. Give it a pulse for 30 seconds until blended well. Serve chilled and fresh. **Nutrition:** *Calories 108	Protein 9 g	Fat 0.2 g	Cholesterol 0.01 mg	Potassium 183 mg	Calcium 57 mg	Fiber 1.2g*	*Preparation Time: 10minutes* *Cooking Time: 0 minutes* *Servings: 1* **Ingredients:** *3/4 cup pineapple sorbet* *1 scoop vanilla protein powder* *1/2 cup water* *2 ice cubes, optional* **Directions:** First, start by putting all the ingredients in a blender jug. Give it a pulse for 30 seconds until blended well. Serve chilled and fresh. *Nutrition:* *Calories 268	Protein 18 g	Fat 4g	Cholesterol 36 mg	Potassium 237 mg	Calcium 160 mg	Fiber 1.4g*

FRUITY SMOOTHIE	MIXED BERRY PROTEIN SMOOTHIE
Preparation Time: 10minutes *Cooking Time: 0 minutes* *Servings: 2* **Ingredients:** *8 oz canned fruits, with juice* *2 scoops vanilla-flavored whey protein powder* *1 cup cold water* *1 cup crushed ice* **Directions:** First, start by putting all the ingredients in a blender jug. Give it a pulse for 30 seconds until blended well. Serve chilled and fresh. **Nutrition:** *Calories 186 | Protein 23 g| Fat 2g | Cholesterol 41 mg | Potassium 282 mg | Calcium 160 mg | Fiber 1.1 g*	*Preparation Time: 10minutes* *Cooking Time: 0 minutes* *Servings: 2* **Ingredients:** *4 oz cold water* *1 cup frozen mixed berries* *2 ice cubes* *1 tsp blueberry essence* *1/2 cup whipped cream topping* *2 scoops whey protein powder* **Directions:** First, start by putting all the ingredients in a blender jug. Give it a pulse for 30 seconds until blended well. Serve chilled and fresh. **Nutritional:** *Calories 104 | Protein 6 g | Fat 4 g | Cholesterol 11 mg | Potassium 141 mg | Calcium 69 mg | Fiber 2.4 g*

PEACH HIGH-PROTEIN SMOOTHIE	STRAWBERRY FRUIT SMOOTHIE
Preparation Time: 10minutes *Cooking Time: 0 minutes* *Servings: 1* **Ingredients:** *1/2 cup ice* *2 tbsp powdered egg whites* *3/4 cup fresh peaches* *1 tbsp sugar* **Directions:** First, start by putting all the ingredients in a blender jug. Give it a pulse for 30 seconds until blended well. Serve chilled and fresh. **Nutrition:** *Calories 132 | Protein 10 g | Fat 0 g | Cholesterol 0 mg | Potassium 353 mg | Calcium 9 mg | Fiber 1.9 g*	*Preparation Time: 10minutes* *Cooking Time: 0 minutes* *Servings: 1* **Ingredients:** *3/4 cup fresh strawberries* *1/2 cup liquid pasteurized egg whites* *1/2 cup ice* *1 tbsp sugar* **Directions:** First, start by putting all the ingredients in a blender jug. Give it a pulse for 30 seconds until blended well. Serve chilled and fresh. **Nutrition:** *Calories 156 | Protein 14 g | Fat 0 g | Cholesterol 0 mg | Potassium 400 mg | Phosphorus 49 mg | Calcium 29 mg | Fiber 2.5 g*

WATERMELON BLISS	CRANBERRY SMOOTHIE
Preparation Time: 10minutes *Cooking Time: 0 minutes* *Servings: 2* **Ingredients:** *2 cups watermelon* *1 medium-sized cucumber, peeled and sliced* *2 mint sprigs, leaves only* *1 celery stalk* *Squeeze of lime juice* **Directions:** First, start by putting all the ingredients in a blender jug. Give it a pulse for 30 seconds until blended well. Serve chilled and fresh. **Nutrition:** *Calories 156	Protein 14 g	Fat 0 g	Cholesterol 0 mg	Potassium 400 mg	Calcium 29 mg	Fiber 2.5g*	*Preparation Time: 10minutes* *Cooking Time: 0 minutes* *Servings: 1* **Ingredients:** *1 cup frozen cranberries* *1 medium cucumber, peeled and sliced* *1 stalk of celery* *Handful of parsley* *Squeeze of lime juice* **Directions:** First, start by putting all the ingredients in a blender jug. Give it a pulse for 30 seconds until blended well. Serve chilled and fresh. **Nutrition:** *Calories 126| Protein 12 g	Fat 0.03 g	Cholesterol 0 mg	Potassium 220 mg	Calcium 19 mg	Fiber 1.4g*

BERRY CUCUMBER SMOOTHIE	RASPBERRY PEACH SMOOTHIE
Preparation Time: 10minutes *Cooking Time: 0 minutes* *Servings: 1* **Ingredients:** *1 medium cucumber, peeled and sliced* *½ cup fresh blueberries* *½ cup fresh or frozen strawberries* *½ cup unsweetened rice milk* *Stevia, to taste* **Directions:** First, start by putting all the ingredients in a blender jug. Give it a pulse for 30 seconds until blended well. Serve chilled and fresh. **Nutrition:** Calories 141 | Protein 10 g | Carbohydrates 15 g | Fat 0 g | Sodium 113 mg | Potassium 230 mg | Phosphorus 129 mg	*Preparation Time: 10minutes* *Cooking Time: 0 minutes* *Servings: 2* **Ingredients:** *1 cup frozen raspberries* *1 medium peach, pit removed, sliced* *½ cup silken tofu* *1 tbsp honey* *1 cup unsweetened vanilla almond milk* **Directions:** First, start by putting all the ingredients in a blender jug. Give it a pulse for 30 seconds until blended well. Serve chilled and fresh. **Nutrition:** Calories 132 | Protein 9 g. | Carbohydrates 14 g | Sodium 112 mg | Potassium 310 mg | Phosphorus 39 mg | Calcium 32 mg

POWER-BOOSTING SMOOTHIE	DISTINCTIVE PINEAPPLE SMOOTHIE
Preparation Time: 5 minutes *Cooking Time: 0 minutes* *Servings: 2* **Ingredients:** *½ cup water* *½ cup non-dairy whipped topping* *2 scoops whey protein powder* *1½ cups frozen blueberries* **Directions:** In a high-speed blender, add all ingredients and pulse till smooth. Transfer into 2 serving glass and serve immediately. **Nutrition:** *Calories 242	Fat 7g	Carbs 23.8g	Protein 23.2g	Potassium (K) 263mg	Sodium (Na) 63mg	Phosphorous 30 mg*	*Preparation Time: 5 minutes* *Cooking Time: 0 minutes* *Servings: 2* **Ingredients:** *¼ cup crushed ice cubes* *2 scoops vanilla whey protein powder* *1 cup water* *1½ cups pineapple* **Directions:** In a high-speed blender, add all ingredients and pulse till smooth. Transfer into 2 serving glass and serve immediately. **Nutrition:** *Calories 117	Fat 2.1g	Carbs 18.2g	Protein 22.7g	Potassium (K) 296mg	Sodium (Na) 81mg	Phosphorous 28 mg*

STRENGTHENING SMOOTHIE BOWL	PINEAPPLE JUICE
Preparation Time: 5 minutes *Cooking Time: 4 minutes* *Servings: 2* **Ingredients:** *¼ cup fresh blueberries* *¼ cup fat-free plain Greek yogurt* *1/3 cup unsweetened almond milk* *2 tbsp of whey protein powder* *2 cups frozen blueberries* **Directions:** In a blender, add blueberries and pulse for about 1 minute. Add almond milk, yogurt and protein powder and pulse till desired consistency. Transfer the mixture into 2 bowls evenly. Serve with the topping of fresh blueberries. **Nutrition:** *Calories 176 | Fat 2.1g | Carbs 27g | Protein 15.1g | Potassium (K) 242mg | Sodium (Na) 72mg | Phosphorous 555.3 mg*	*Preparation Time: 5 minutes* *Cooking Time: 0 minutes* *Servings: 2* **Ingredients:** *½ cup canned pineapple* *1 cup water* **Direction:** Blend all ingredients and serve over ice. **Nutrition:** *Calories 135 | Protein 0 g| Carbs 0 g | Fat 0 g | Sodium (Na) 0 mg | Potassium (K) 180 mg | Phosphorus 8 mg*

GRAPEFRUIT SORBET	APPLE AND BLUEBERRY CRISP
Preparation time: 10 minutes *Cooking time: 5 minutes* *Servings: 6* **Ingredients** *½ cup sugar* *¼ cup water* *1 fresh thyme sprig* *For the sorbet* *Juice of 6 pink grapefruit* *¼ cup thyme simple syrup* *To make the thyme simple syrup* *In a small saucepan, combine the sugar, water, and thyme. Bring to a boil, turn off the heat, and refrigerate, thyme sprig included, until cold. Strain the thyme sprig from the syrup.* *To make the sorbet* **Directions:** In a blender, combine the grapefruit juice and ¼ cup of simple syrup, and process. Transfer to an airtight container and freeze for 3 to 4 hours, until firm. Serve. Substitution tip: Try this with other citrus fruits, such as oranges, lemons, or limes, for an equally delicious treat. **Nutrition:** *Calories 117 | Fat 2.1g | Carbs 18.2g | Protein 22.7g | Potassium (K) 296mg | Sodium (Na) 81mg | Phosphorous 28 mg*	***Preparation time**: 1 hour 10 minutes* ***Cooking time**: 1 hour* ***Serving**: 8* **Ingredients:** *Crisp* *1/4 cup of brown sugar* *1 1/4 cups quick cooking rolled oats* *6 tbsp non-hydrogenated melted margarine* *1/4 cup all-purpose flour (unbleached)* **Filling:** *2 tbsp cornstarch* *1/2 cup of brown sugar* *2 cups chopped or grated apples* *4 cups frozen or fresh blueberries (not thawed)* *1 tbsp fresh lemon juice* *1 tbsp melted margarine* **Directions:** Preheat the oven to 350°F with the rack in the middle position. Pour all the dry ingredients into a bowl, then the butter and stir until it is moistened. Set the mixture aside. In an 8-inch (20-cm) square baking dish, mix the cornstarch and brown sugar. Add lemon juice and the rest of the fruits. Toss to blend the mixture. Add the crisp mixture, then bake until the crisp turns golden brown (or for 55 minutes to 1 hour). You can either serve cold or warm. **Nutrition:** *Calories 127 | Fat 2.1g | Carbs 18.2g | Protein 22.7g | Potassium (K) 256mg | Sodium (Na) 61mg | Phosphorous 28 mg*

MINI PINEAPPLE UPSIDE DOWN CAKES

Preparation time: 50 minutes
Cooking time: 50 minutes
Serving: 12
Ingredients:
3 tbsp melted unsalted butter
12 canned unsweetened pineapple slices
1/3 cup packed brown sugar
2/3 cup sugar
6 fresh cherries cut into halves and pitted
3 tbsp canola oil
2/3 cup milk (fat-free)
½ tbsp lemon juice
1 large egg
1-1/3 cups cake flour
1/4 tbsp vanilla extract
1/4 tsp salt
1-1/4 tsp baking powder
Directions:
Coat 12 serving muffin pan with butter or you could use a square baking pan.
Sprinkle little brown sugar into each of the sections. Crush 1 pineapple slice into each section to take the shape of the cup. Place 1 half cherry in the center of the pineapple with the cut side facing up.
Get a large bowl and beat the egg, milk, and the extracts until it is evenly blended.
Beat the flour, salt, and baking powder into sugar mixture until it is well blended to attain homogeneity and pour it into the batter prepared in the muffin pan.
Bake at 350°s until a toothpick sinks in and comes out clean (or for 35-40 minutes). Invert the muffin pan immediately and allow the cooked cakes to drop onto a serving plate. (If necessary, you can use a small spatula or butter knife to release them from the pan gently.) Serve warm.
Nutrition:
Calories 119 | Fat 2.1g | Carbs 16.2g | Protein 22.7g | Potassium (K) 296mg | Sodium (Na) 81mg | Phosphorous 28 mg

FRESH FRUIT COMPOTE

Preparation time: 10 minutes
Cooking time: 10 minutes
Serving: 8
Ingredients:
1/2 cup fresh or frozen blackberries
1/2 cup fresh or frozen strawberries
1/2 cup pared peaches (diced)
1/2 cup fresh or frozen blueberries
1/2 cup orange juice (unsweetened)
1/4 cup frozen or fresh red raspberries (not thawed and sweetened)
1 banana (diced, bite-size pieces)
1 apple (diced, bite-size pieces)
Directions:
Pour some orange juice into a large container.
Pour all the listed ingredients.
Mix gently.
If you're using frozen fruit, let it thaw for 4 hours at ambient temperature.

Nutrition:
Calories 117 | Fat 2.1g | Carbs 18.2g | Protein 22.7g | Potassium (K) 296mg | Sodium (Na) 81mg | Phosphorous 18 mg

APPLE CINNAMON FARFEL KUGEL

Preparation time: 45 minutes
Cooking time: 45 minutes
Serving: 6
Ingredients:
3 egg (large) whites
1 cup hot water
1/4 cup sugar
1 cup Matzo farfel
1 tbsp ground cinnamon
2 large apples
1/2 cup pineapple chunks
Directions:
Preheat the oven to about 375°F.
Peel, cut and shred the apples.
Get an 8" x 8" baking dish and spray it with cooking spray.
In another large bowl, mix the farfel and hot water.
Add the apples, cinnamon, and sugar.
Beat the egg whites and fold the egg whites.
Pour the drained pineapple chunks and mix together.
Transfer the mixture into the already prepared baking dish and sprinkle the top with additional cinnamon.
Bake for about 45 minutes.
Nutrition:
Calories 137 | Fat 2.1g | Carbs 18.2g | Protein 12.7g | Potassium (K) 296mg | Sodium (Na) 71mg | Phosphorous 28 mg

CREPES WITH FROZEN BERRIES

Preparation time: 25 minutes
Cooking time: 25 minutes
Serving: 4
Ingredients:
2 egg whites
1/2 cup all-purpose white flour
1 tbsp canola oil
1/2 cup nonfat milk
1 tbsp powdered sugar
1/2 cup mixed frozen berries
Directions:
Allow the frozen berries to thaw then drain the mixed berries.
In a large bowl, whisk the egg white, flour, milk, salt, and oil together until it is smooth.
Coat a skillet lightly with cooking spray and adjust the oven to medium heat. Pour about 1/4 cup of batter into the prepared skillet. Tilt the pan continuously in a circular motion to ensure the batter spread to the edges. Cook for about 2 minutes or until the bottom is light brown.
Turn the crepe and add 2 tablespoons of mixed berries to the center of the crepe, then cook an additional 2 minutes. With a spatula, fold the crepe in half and transfer it to a serving plate. Sprinkle with sugar or other confectionery. Once, it is to your liking, it is ready to serve.
Nutrition:
Calories 117 | Fat 2.1g | Carbs 18.2g | Protein 22.7g | Potassium (K) 296mg | Sodium (Na) 81mg | Phosphorous 28 mg

TROPICAL GRANITA	ICE CREAM SANDWICHES
Preparation time: 5 minutes *Cooking time: 0 minutes* *Servings: 4* **Ingredients**: *1 cup fresh or frozen pineapple chunks* *½ cup fresh or frozen mango chunks* *2 cups orange juice* *Juice of 1 lime* *Fresh mint, for garnish* **Directions**: In a blender, combine the pineapple, mango, orange juice, and lime juice. Process until smooth, and transfer to a freezer-safe dish. Freeze for 2 hours. Use a fork to break the mixture apart into smaller granular pieces. Serve garnished with pieces of torn mint leaves. Cooking tip: If you freeze the granita too long, it will become solid. Let it sit out for about 20 minutes until it is breakable, and separate it into a few chunks, then pulse in a blender until its consistency resembles shaved ice. **Nutrition**: *Calories 107 | Fat 2.1g | Carbs 18.2g | Protein 12.7g | Potassium (K) 226mg | Sodium (Na) 81mg | Phosphorous 28 mg*	*Preparation time: 7 minutes* *Cooking time: 0 minutes* *Serving: 10* **Ingredients**: *20 tbsp cool whip (non-dairy)* *10 plain graham crackers* *Directions:* *Break the graham crackers into halves.* *Sprinkle 2 teaspoons of cool whip on one half.* *Place the other half of the cracker on the one that was sprinkled.* *Place them on a tray and freeze it for a couple of hours.* *Once it is frozen, wrap each of the sandwiches with Saran Wrap.* **Nutrition:** *Calories 117 | Fat 2.1g | Carbs 18.2g | Protein 22.7g | Potassium (K) 296mg | Sodium (Na) 81mg | Phosphorous 28 mg*

BLUEBERRY BURST	PEACH ICED-TEA
Preparation time:5 minutes *Cooking time: 0 minutes* *Servings: 2* **Ingredients:** *1 cup chopped collard greens* *1 cup unsweetened rice milk* *1 tbsp. almond butter* *1 cup blueberries* *3 ice cubes* **Directions:** Combine everything in a blender until smooth. Pour into 2 glasses and serve. **Nutrition:** *Calories 131 | Sodium (Na) 60 mg | Protein 3 g | Potassium 146 mg | Phosphorus 51 mg | Carbs 4 g, | Fat 0 g*	*Preparation time: 15 minutes* *Cooking time: 0 minutes* *Servings: 2* **Ingredients:** *1 lemon* *1 cup sliced canned peaches* *1 tbsp. loose black* **Directions:** Boil a pot of water and add the peach slices. Simmer for 10 minutes before turning off the heat. Add the loose tea leaves and allow to steep for 5-7 minutes. Pour liquid through a sieve or tea strainer. Enjoy hot. **Nutrition:** *Calories 74 | Protein 0 g Carbs 15 g | Fat 0 g | Sodium (Na) 5 mg | Potassium (K) 15 mg | Phosphorus 14 mg*

LEMON BOOST

Preparation time: 5 minutes
Cooking time: 0 minutes
Servings: 2
Ingredients:
1 tsp. cinnamon
2 tbsps. stevia
1 juiced lemon
2 pasteurized liquid egg whites
Directions:
Combine all ingredients in a blender until smooth.
Garnish with a slice of lemon and serve over ice!
Nutrition:
Calories 30 | Protein 3 g | Carbs 3 g | Fat 1 g |
Sodium (Na)55 mg | Potassium (K) 86 mg |
Phosphorus 10 mg

Chapter 11: Snacks and Side

FLUFFY MOCK PANCAKES	MIXES OF SNACK
Preparation time: 5 minutes *Cooking time: 10 minutes* *Servings: 2* **Ingredients** *1 egg* *1 cup ricotta cheese* *1 teaspoon cinnamon* *2 tablespoons honey, add more if needed* **Directions** Using a blender, put together egg, honey, cinnamon, and ricotta cheese. Process until all ingredients are well combined. Pour an equal amount of the blended mixture into the pan. Cook each pancake for 4 minutes on both sides. Serve. **Nutrition:** *Calories: 188.1 kcal | Total fat: 14.5 g |Saturated fat: 4.5 g | Cholesterol: 139.5 mg | Sodium: 175.5 mg | Total carbs: 5.5 g | Fiber: 2.8 g | Sugar: 0.9 g | Protein: 8.5 g*	*Preparation time: 10 minutes* *Cooking time: 1 hours and 15 minutes* *Servings: 4* **Ingredients** *6 cup margarine* *2 tablespoon worcestershire sauce* *1 ½ tablespoon spice salt* *¾ cup garlic powder* *½ teaspoon onion powder* *3 cups crispi* *3 cups cheerios* *3 cups corn flakes* *1 cup kixe* *1 cup pretzels* *1 cup broken bagel chips into 1-inch pieces* **Directions** Preheat the oven to 250f (120c) Melt the margarine in a pan. Stir in the seasoning. Gradually add the ingredients remaining by mixing so that the coating is uniform. Cook 1 hour, stirring every 15 minutes. Spread on paper towels to let cool. Store in a tightly-closed container. **Nutrition:** *Calories: 200 kcal | Total fat: 9 g | Saturated fat: 3.5 g | Cholesterol: 0 mg | Sodium: 3.5 mg | Total carbs: 27 g | Fiber: 2 g | Sugar: 0 g | Protein: 3 g*

CRANBERRY DIP WITH FRESH FRUIT

Preparation time: 10 minutes
Cooking time: 0 minutes
Servings: 8
Ingredients
8-ounce sour cream
1/2 cup whole berry cranberry sauce
1/4 teaspoon nutmeg
1/4 teaspoon ground ginger
4 cups fresh pineapple, peeled, cubed
4 medium apples, peeled, cored and cubed
4 medium pears, peeled, cored and cubed
1 teaspoon lemon juice
Directions
Start by adding cranberry sauce, sour cream, ginger, and nutmeg to a food processor.
Blend the mixture until its smooth then transfer it to a bowl.
Toss the pineapple, with pears, apples, and lemon juice in a salad bowl.
Thread the fruits onto mini skewers.
Serve them with the sauce.

Nutrition:
Calories 70 | Protein 0 g | Carbohydrates 13 g | Fat 2 g | Cholesterol 4 mg | Sodium 8 mg | Potassium 101 mg | Phosphorus 15 mg | Calcium 17 mg | Fiber 1.5 g

CUCUMBERS WITH SOUR CREAM

Preparation time: 10 minutes
Cooking time: 0 minutes
Servings: 4
Ingredients
2 medium cucumbers, peeled and sliced thinly
1/2 medium sweet onion, sliced
1/4 cup white wine vinegar
1 tablespoon canola oil
1/8 teaspoon black pepper
1/2 cup reduced-fat sour cream
Directions
Toss in cucumber, onion, and all other ingredients in a medium-size bowl.
Mix well and refrigerate for 2 hours.
Toss again and serve to enjoy.

Nutrition:
Calories 64 | Protein 1 g | Carbohydrates 4 g | Fat 5 g | Cholesterol 3 mg |Sodium 72 mg| Potassium 113 mg | Phosphorus 24 mg | Calcium 21 mg | Fiber 0.8 g

SWEET SAVORY MEATBALLS

Preparation time: 10 minutes
Cooking time: 20 minutes
Servings: 12
Ingredients
1-pound ground turkey
1 large egg
1/4 cup bread crumbs
2 tablespoon onion, finely chopped
1 teaspoon garlic powder
1/2 teaspoon black pepper
1/4 cup canola oil
6-ounce grape jelly
1/4 cup chili sauce
Directions
Place all ingredients except chili sauce and jelly in a large mixing bowl.
Mix well until evenly mixed then make small balls out of this mixture.
It will make about 48 meatballs. Spread them out on a greased pan on a stovetop.
Cook them over medium heat until brown on all the sides.
Mix chili sauce with jelly in a microwave-safe bowl and heat it for 2 minutes in the microwave.
Pour this chili sauce mixture onto the meatballs in the pan.
Transfer the meatballs in the pan to the preheated oven.
Bake the meatballs for 20 minutes in an oven at 375 degrees f.
Serve fresh and warm.
Nutrition:
Calories 127. Protein 9 g | Carbohydrates 14 g | Fat 4 g | Cholesterol 41 mg | Sodium 129 mg | Potassium 148 mg | Phosphorus 89 mg | Calcium 15 mg | Fiber 0.2 g

SPICY CORN BREAD

Preparation time: 10 minutes
Cooking time: 30 minutes
Servings: 8
Ingredients
1 cup all-purpose white flour
1 cup plain cornmeal
1 tablespoon sugar
2 teaspoon baking powder
1 teaspoon chili powder
1/4 teaspoon black pepper
1 cup rice milk, unenriched
1 egg
1 egg white
2 tablespoon canola oil
1/2 cup scallions, finely chopped
1/4 cup carrots, finely grated
1 garlic clove, minced
Directions
Preheat your oven to 400 degrees f.
Now start by mixing the flour with baking powder, sugar, cornmeal, pepper and chili powder in a mixing bowl.
Stir in oil, milk, egg white, and egg.
Mix well until it's smooth then stir in carrots, garlic, and scallions.
Stir well then spread the batter in an 8-inch baking pan greased with cooking spray.
Bake for 30 minutes until golden brown.
Slice and serve fresh.
Nutrition:
Calories 188 | Protein 5 g | Carbohydrates 31 g | Fat 5 g | Cholesterol 26 mg | Sodium 155 mg | Potassium 100 mg | Phosphorus 81 mg | Calcium 84 mg | Fiber 2 g

SWEET AND SPICY TORTILLA CHIPS	ADDICTIVE PRETZELS
Preparation time: 10 minutes *Cooking time: 8 minutes* *Servings: 6* **Ingredients** *1/4 cup butter* *1 teaspoon brown sugar* *1/2 teaspoon ground chili powder* *1/2 teaspoon garlic powder* *1/2 teaspoon ground cumin* *1/4 teaspoon ground cayenne pepper* *6 flour tortillas, 6" size* **Directions** Preheat oven to 425 degrees f. Grease a baking sheet with cooking spray. Add all spices, brown sugar, and melted butter to a small bowl. Mix well and set this mixture aside. Slice the tortillas into 8 wedges and brush them with the sugar mixture. Spread them on the baking sheet and bake them for 8 minutes. Serve fresh. **Nutrition:** *Calories 115 | Protein 2 g | Carbohydrates 11 g | Fat 7 g | Cholesterol 15 mg | Sodium 156 mg | Potassium 42 mg | Phosphorus 44 mg | Calcium 31 mg | Fiber 0.6 g*	*Preparation time: 10 minutes* *Cooking time: 1 hour* *Servings: 6* **Ingredients** *32-ounce bag unsalted pretzels* *1 cup canola oil* *2 tablespoon seasoning mix* *3 teaspoon garlic powder* *3 teaspoon dried dill weed* **Directions** Preheat oven to 175 degrees f. Place the pretzels on a cooking sheet and break them into pieces. Mix garlic powder and dill in a bowl and reserve half of the mixture. Mix the remaining half with seasoning mix and ¾ cup of canola oil. Pour this oil over the pretzels and brush them liberally Bake the pieces for 1 hour then flip them to bake for another 15 minutes. Allow them to cool then sprinkle the remaining dill mixture and drizzle more oil on top. Serve fresh and warm. **Nutrition:** Calories 184 | Protein 2 g | Carbohydrates 22 g | Fat 8 g | Cholesterol 0 mg | Sodium 60 mg | Potassium 43 mg | Phosphorus 28 mg | Calcium 2 mg | Fiber 1.0 g

SHRIMP SPREAD WITH CRACKERS

Preparation time: 10 minutes
Cooking time: 0 minutes
Servings: 6
Ingredients
1/4 cup light cream cheese
2 1/2-ounce cooked, shelled shrimp, minced
1 tablespoon no-salt-added ketchup
1/4 teaspoon hot sauce
1 teaspoon worcestershire sauce
1/2 teaspoon herb seasoning blend
24 matzo cracker miniatures
1 tablespoon parsley
Directions
Start by tossing the minced shrimp with cream cheese in a bowl.
Stir in worcestershire sauce, hot sauce, herb seasoning, and ketchup.
Mix well and garnish with minced parsley.
Serve the spread with the crackers.

Nutrition:
Calories 57 | Protein 3 g | Carbohydrates 7 g | Fat 1 g | Cholesterol 21 mg | Sodium 69 mg | Potassium 54 mg | Phosphorus 30 mg | Calcium 15 mg | Fiber 0.2 g

BUFFALO CHICKEN DIP

Preparation time: 10 minutes
Cooking time: 3 hours
Servings: 4
Ingredients
4-ounce cream cheese
1/2 cup bottled roasted red peppers
1 cup reduced-fat sour cream
4 teaspoon hot pepper sauce
2 cups cooked, shredded chicken
Directions
Blend half cup of drained red peppers in a food processor until smooth.
Now, thoroughly mix cream cheese, and sour cream with the pureed peppers in a bowl.
Stir in shredded chicken and hot sauce then transfer the mixture to a slow cooker.
Cook for 3 hours on low heat.
Serve warm with celery, carrots, cauliflower, and cucumber.

Nutrition:
Calories 73 | Protein 5 g | Carbohydrates 2 g | Fat 5 g | Cholesterol 25 mg | Sodium 66 mg | Potassium 81 mg | Phosphorus 47 mg | Calcium 31 mg | Fiber 0 g

CHICKEN PEPPER BACON WRAPS

Preparation time: 10 minutes
Cooking time: 15 minutes
Servings: 4
Ingredients
1 medium onion, chopped
12 strips bacon, halved
12 fresh jalapenos peppers
12 fresh banana peppers
2 pounds boneless, skinless chicken breast
Directions
How to prepare:
Grease a grill rack with cooking spray and preheat the grill on low heat.
Slice the peppers in half lengthwise then remove their seeds.
Dice the chicken into small pieces and divide them into each pepper.
Now spread the chopped onion over the chicken in the peppers.
Wrap the bacon strips around the stuffed peppers.
Place these wrapped peppers in the grill and cook them for 15 minutes.
Serve fresh and warm.

Nutrition:
Calories 71. Protein 10 g | Carbohydrates 1 g | Fat 3 g | Cholesterol 26 mg | Sodium 96 mg | Potassium 147 mg | Phosphorus 84 mg | Calcium 9 mg | Fiber 0.8 g

GARLIC OYSTER CRACKERS.

Preparation time: 10 minutes
Cooking time: 45 minutes
Servings: 4
Ingredients
1/2 cup butter-flavored popcorn oil
1 tablespoon garlic powder
7 cups oyster crackers
2 teaspoon dried dill weed
Directions
How to prepare:
Preheat oven to 250 degrees f.
Mix garlic powder with oil in a large bowl.
Toss in crackers and mix well to coat evenly.
Sprinkle the dill weed over the crackers and toss well again.
Spread the crackers on the baking sheet and bake them for 45 minutes.
Toss them every 15 minutes.
Serve fresh.
Nutrition:
Calories 118 | Protein 2 g | Carbohydrates 12 g | Fat 7 g | Cholesterol 0 mg | Sodium 166 mg | Potassium 21 mg | Phosphorus 15 mg | Calcium 4 mg | Fiber 3 g

LIME CILANTRO RICE	SPANISH RICE
Preparation time: 5 minutes *Cooking time: 20 minutes* *Servings: 2* **Ingredients** *White rice – .75 cup* *Water – 1.5 cups* *Olive oil – 1.5 tablespoons* *Bay leaf, ground - .25 teaspoon* *Lime juice – 1 tablespoon* *Lemon juice – 1 tablespoon* *Lime zest - .25 teaspoon* *Cilantro, chopped - .25 cup* **Directions** Place the white rice and water in a medium-sized saucepan and bring it to a boil over medium heat. Simmer and cover the pot with a lid, allowing it to cook until all water has been absorbed about eighteen to twenty minutes. Stir in the ground bay leaf, olive oil, lime juice, lemon juice, lime zest, and cilantro after cooking. You want to do this with a fork, preferably, as this will fluff the rice rather than causing it to compact. Serve while warm. **Nutrition:** *Calories in individual servings: 363	Protein grams: 5	Phosphorus milligrams: 74	Potassium milligrams: 86	Sodium milligrams: 5	Fat grams: 10	Total carbohydrates grams: 60	Net carbohydrates grams: 58*	*Preparation time: 5 minutes* *Cooking time: 20 minutes* *Servings: 2* **Ingredients** *White rice – .75 cup* *Chicken broth, low sodium– 1.5 cups* *Onion dehydrated flakes – 2 tablespoons* *Garlic, minced – 2 cloves* *Lemon juice – 1 tablespoon* *Cumin, ground - .25 teaspoon* *Chili powder - .5 teaspoon* *Oregano, dried - .5 teaspoon* *Black pepper, ground - .25 teaspoon* *Cilantro, chopped – 3 tablespoons* **Directions** Place the rice, chicken broth, onion flakes, and minced garlic in a medium-sized saucepan. Bring the chicken broth and the rice to a boil over medium heat, and then reduce the heat to a light simmer, cover it with a lid, and allow it to cook until the liquid has all been absorbed about eighteen to twenty minutes. Use a fork to fluff the rice mix in the lemon juice, cumin, chili powder, oregano, black pepper, and cilantro. Once combined, serve the rice while still warm. **Nutrition:** *Calories in individual servings: 303	Protein grams: 6	Phosphorus milligrams: 104	Potassium milligrams: 197	Sodium milligrams: 57	Fat grams: 1	Total carbohydrates grams: 65	Net carbohydrates grams: 63*

Chapter 12: Soups

LAMB STEW	SAUSAGE & EGG SOUP
Preparation Time: 30 minutes *Cooking Time: 1 hour and 40 minutes* *Servings: 6* **Ingredients:** *1 lb. boneless lamb shoulder, trimmed and cubes* *Black pepper to taste* *1/4 cup all-purpose flour* *1 tablespoon olive oil* *1 onion, chopped* *3 garlic cloves, chopped* *1/2 cup tomato sauce* *2 cups low-sodium beef broth* *1 teaspoon dried thyme* *2 parsnips, sliced* *2 carrots, sliced* *1 cup frozen peas* **Directions:** Season the lamb with pepper Coat it evenly with flour. Pour oil in a pot over medium heat. Cook the lamb and then set aside. Add onion to the pot. Cook for 2 minutes. Add garlic and sauté for 30 seconds. Pour in the broth to deglaze the pot. Add the tomato sauce and thyme. Put the lamb back to the pot. Bring to a boil and then simmer for 1 hour. Add parsnips and carrots. Cook for 30 minutes. Add green peas and cook for 5 minutes. **Nutrition:** *Calories: 156;	Total Fat: 11g;	Cholesterol: 26mg;* *| Carbohydrates: 17g;	Fiber: 3g	Protein: 7g |* *Phosphorus: 115mg	Potassium: 567mg	Sodium: 148mg*	*Preparation Time: 15 minutes* *Cooking Time: 30 minutes* *Servings: 4* **Ingredients:** *1/2 lb. ground beef* *Black pepper* *1/2 teaspoon ground sage* *1/2 teaspoon garlic powder* *1/2 teaspoon dried basil* *4 slices bread (one day old), cubed* *2 tablespoons olive oil* *1 tablespoon herb seasoning blend* *2 garlic cloves, minced* *3 cups low-sodium chicken broth* *1 cup water* *4 tablespoons fresh parsley* *4 eggs* *2 tablespoons Parmesan cheese, grated* **Directions:** Preheat your oven to 375 degrees F. Mix the first five **Ingredients** to make the sausage. Toss bread cubes in oil and seasoning blend. Bake in the oven for 8 minutes. Set aside. Cook the sausage in a pan over medium heat. Cook the garlic in the sausage drippings for 2 minutes. Stir in the broth, water and parsley. Bring to a boil and then simmer for 10 minutes. Pour into serving bowls and top with baked bread, egg and sausage. **Nutrition:** *Calories: 196	Fat: 11g	Cholesterol: 26mg |* *Carbohydrates: 17g| Fiber: 3g	Protein: 7g |* *Phosphorus: 125mg	Potassium: 537mg	Sodium: 148mg*

SPRING VEGGIE SOUP	SEAFOOD CHOWDER WITH CORN
Preparation Time: 20 minutes *Cooking Time: 45 minutes* *Servings: 5* **Ingredients**: *2 tablespoons olive oil* *1/2 cup onion, diced* *1/2 cup mushrooms, sliced* *1/8 cup celery, chopped* *1 tomato, diced* *1/2 cup carrots, diced* *1 cup green beans, trimmed* *1/2 cup frozen corn* *1 teaspoon garlic powder* *1 teaspoon dried oregano leaves* *4 cups low-sodium vegetable broth* **Directions:** In a pot, pour the olive oil and cook the onion and celery for 2 minutes. Add the rest of the **Ingredients**. Bring to a boil. Reduce heat and simmer for 45 minutes. **Nutrition:** *Calories: 136	Total Fat: 11g |Cholesterol: 26mg	Carbohydrates: 17g	Fiber: 3g	Protein: 7g	Phosphorus: 125mg	Potassium: 527mg	Sodium: 138mg*	*Preparation Time: 15 minutes* *Cooking Time: 20 minutes* *Servings: 10* **Ingredients**: *1 tablespoon butter (unsalted)* *1 cup onion, chopped* *½ cup red bell pepper, chopped* *½ cup green bell pepper, chopped* *¼ cup celery, chopped* *1 tablespoon all-purpose white flour* *14 oz. low-sodium chicken broth* *2 cups non-dairy creamer* *6 oz. almond milk* *10 oz. crab flakes* *2 cups corn kernels* *½ teaspoon paprika* *Black pepper to taste* **Directions:** In a pan over medium heat, melt the butter and cook the onion, bell peppers and celery for 4 minutes. Stir in the flour and cook for 2 minutes. Add the broth and bring to a boil. Add the rest of the **Ingredients**. Stir occasionally, and cook for 5 minutes. **Nutrition:** *Calories: 156	Fat: 11g	Cholesterol: 26mg	Carbohydrates: 17g	Fiber: 3g	Protein: 7g	Phosphorus: 125mg	Potassium: 527mg	Sodium: 128mg*

TACO SOUP

Preparation Time: 30 minutes
Cooking Time: 7 hours
Servings: 10
Ingredients:
1 lb. chicken breast (boneless, skinless)
15 oz. canned red kidney beans, rinsed and drained
15 oz. low-sodium white corn, rinsed and drained
15 oz. canned yellow hominy, rinsed and drained
1 cup canned tomatoes with green chilies,diced
1/2 cup onion, chopped
1/2 cup green bell peppers, chopped
1 clove garlic, chopped
1 jalapeno, chopped
1 tablespoon low-sodium taco seasoning
2 cups low-sodium chicken broth
Directions:
Put chicken in the slow cooker.
Top with the rest of the **Ingredients**.
Cook on high for 1 hour.
Set to low and cook for 6 hours.
Shred chicken and serve with the soup.
Nutrition:
Calories: 86 | Fat: 18g | Cholesterol: 26mg |
Carbohydrates: 17g | Fiber: 3g | Protein: 7g |
Phosphorus: 125mg | Potassium: 517mg | Sodium:
248mg

EASY LOW-SODIUM CHICKEN BROTH

Preparation Time: 10 minutes
Cooking Time: 4 hours
Ingredients:
2 pounds skinless whole chicken, cut into pieces
4 garlic cloves, lightly crushed
2 celery stalks, with greens, roughly chopped
2 carrots, roughly chopped
1 sweet onion, cut into quarters
10 peppercorns
4 fresh thyme sprigs
2 bay leaves
Water
Directions:
In a large stockpot, place the chicken, garlic, celery, carrots, onion, peppercorns, thyme, and and bay leaves, and cover with water by about 3 inches.
Bring the water to a boil over high heat, then reduce the heat to medium-low and simmer, uncovered, for about 4 hours
Skim off any foam on top of the stock, and pour the stock through a fine-mesh sieve.
Pick off all the usable chicken meat for another recipe, discard the bones and other solids, and allow the stock to cool for about 30 minutes before transferring it to sealable containers.
Store the stock in the refrigerator for up to 1 week, or in the freezer for up to 2 months.
Ingredient tip: If you enjoy making roast chicken for dinner, keep the carcasses after you have stripped off all the meat, and store the bones in a resealable bag in the freezer. Once you have two or three bags saved, you can use the carcasses to make this stock.
Nutrition:
Calories: 186 | Fat: 11g | Cholesterol: 26mg |
Carbohydrates: 17g | Fiber: 3g | Protein: 7g |
Phosphorus: 125mg | Potassium: 557mg | Sodium:
148mg

PESTO GREEN VEGETABLE SOUP

Preparation Time: 10 minutes
Cooking Time: 15 minutes
Servings: 6
Ingredients:
2 teaspoons olive oil
1 leek, white and light green parts, sliced and washed thoroughly
2 celery stalks, diced
1 teaspoon minced garlic
2 cups sodium-free chicken stock
1 cup chopped snow peas
1 cup shredded spinach
1 tablespoon chopped fresh thyme
Juice and zest of ½ lemons
¼ teaspoons freshly ground black pepper
1 tablespoon Basil Pesto
Directions:
In a large saucepan over medium-high heat, heat the olive oil.
Add the leek, celery, and garlic, and sauté until tender, about 3 minutes.
Stir in the stock, and bring to a boil.
Stir in the snow peas, spinach, and thyme, and simmer for about 5 minutes.
Remove the pan from the heat, and stir in the lemon juice, lemon zest, pepper, and pesto.
Serve immediately.
Low-sodium tip: Commercially prepared pesto has about 145 mg of sodium per tablespoon. Making your own pesto from fresh basil leaves, olive oil, fresh garlic, and freshly ground black pepper allows you to decrease that sodium amount per tablespoon down to zero.
Nutrition:
Calories: 136 | Fat: 11g | Cholesterol: 16mg | Carbohydrates: 17g | Fiber: 3g | Protein: 7g | Phosphorus: 125mg | Potassium: 527mg | Sodium: 148mg

VEGETABLE MINESTRONE

Preparation Time: 20 minutes
Cooking Time: 20 minutes
Servings: 6
Ingredients:
1 teaspoon olive oil
½ sweet onion, chopped
1 celery stalk, diced
1 teaspoon minced garlic
2 cups sodium-free chicken stock
2 medium tomatoes, chopped
1 zucchini, diced
½ cup shredded stemmed kale
Freshly ground black pepper
1-ounce grated Parmesan cheese

Directions:
In a large saucepan over medium-high heat, heat the olive oil.
Add the onion, celery, and garlic, and sauté until softened, about 5 minutes.
Stir in the stock, tomatoes, and zucchini, and bring to a boil.
Reduce the heat to low, and simmer for 15 minutes.
Stir in the kale, and season with pepper.
Garnish with the Parmesan cheese, and serve.
Low-sodium tip: There is not much sodium in this recipe, but you could cut it further by omitting the Parmesan cheese. One tablespoon of Parmesan has about 80 mg of sodium.
Nutrition:
Calories: 86 | Total Fat: 11g | Cholesterol: 16mg | Carbohydrates: 17g | Fiber: 3g | Protein: 7g | Phosphorus: 115mg | Potassium: 257mg | Sodium: 248mg

CREAMY BROCCOLI SOUP	CURRIED CARROT AND BEET SOUP
Preparation Time: 10 minutes *Cooking Time: 15 minutes* *Servings: 4* **Ingredients:** *1 teaspoon extra-virgin olive oil* *½ sweet onion, roughly chopped* *2 cups chopped broccoli* *4 cups low-sodium vegetable broth* *Freshly ground black pepper* *1 cup Homemade Rice Milk or unsweetened store-bought rice milk* *¼ cup grated Parmesan cheese* **Directions:** In a medium saucepan over medium-high heat, heat the olive oil. Add the onion and cook for 3 to 5 minutes, until it begins to soften. Add the broccoli and broth, and season with pepper. Bring to a boil, reduce the heat, and simmer uncovered for 10 minutes, until the broccoli is just tender but still bright green. Transfer the soup mixture to a blender. Add the rice milk, and process until smooth. Return to the saucepan, stir in the Parmesan cheese, and serve. Substitution tip: You can use this recipe to make several varieties of green soups. Experiment by substituting spinach, a mix of arugula and kale, or micro greens, for a twist on the ordinary that suits your tastes. **Nutrition:** *Calories: 126 | Total Fat: 11g | Cholesterol: 26mg |Carbohydrates: 17g | Fiber: 3g| Protein: 7g| Phosphorus: 115mg | Potassium: 337mg | Sodium: 128mg*	*Preparation Time: 10 minutes* *Cooking Time: 50 minutes* *Servings: 4* **Ingredients:** *1 large red beet* *5 carrots, chopped* *1 tablespoon curry powder* *3 cups Homemade Rice Milk or unsweetened store-bought rice milk* *Freshly ground black pepper* *Yogurt, for serving* **Directions:** Preheat the oven to 400°F. Wrap the beet in aluminum foil and roast for 45 minutes, until the vegetable is tender when pierced with a fork. Remove from the oven and let cool. In a saucepan, add the carrots and cover with water. Bring to a boil, reduce the heat, cover, and simmer for 10 minutes, until tender. Transfer the carrots and beet to a food processor and process until smooth. Add the curry powder and rice milk. Season it with pepper. Serve topped with a dollop of yogurt. Substitution tip: Carrots are high in potassium. If you need to reduce your potassium further, use 2 carrots instead of 5. The soup will be a little thinner but still have a carrot flavor and just 322mg of potassium. **Nutrition:** *Calories: 186 | Fat: 11g | Cholesterol: 26mg | Carbohydrates: 17g | Fiber: 3g | Protein: 7g | Phosphorus: 225mg | Potassium: 357mg | Sodium: 248mg*

GOLDEN BEET SOUP

Preparation Time: 10 minutes
Cooking Time: 35 minutes
Servings: 4

Ingredients:

3 tablespoons unsalted butter
4 golden beets cut into ½-inch cubes
½ sweet onion, chopped
1-inch piece ginger, minced
Zest and juice of 1 lemon
4 cups Simple Chicken Broth or low-sodium store-bought chicken stock
Freshly ground black pepper
¼ cup pomegranate seeds, for serving
¼ cup crème fraîche, for serving (see Substitution tip)
10 sage leaves, for serving

Directions:

In a medium saucepan over medium heat, melt the butter.

Add the beets, onion, ginger, and lemon zest, and cover. Cook, stirring occasionally, for 15 minutes.

Add the broth, and continue to cook for 20 more minutes, until the beets are very tender.

In batches, transfer the soup to a blender and purée, or use an immersion blender.

Return the soup to the saucepan, and season with the pepper and lemon juice.

Serve topped with the pomegranate seeds, crème fraîche, and sage leaves.

Substitution tip: You can buy crème fraîche at many grocery stores, or make your own. If you don't have crème fraîche, a dollop of whole-milk yogurt is a fine substitute.

Nutrition:

Calories: 186 | Total Fat: 11g | Cholesterol: 26mg | Carbohydrates: 17g | Fiber: 3g | Protein: 7g | Phosphorus: 125mg | Potassium: 557mg | Sodium: 148mg

ASPARAGUS LEMON SOUP

Preparation Time: 10 minutes
Cooking Time: 25 minutes
Servings: 4

Ingredients:

1 pound asparagus
2 tablespoons extra-virgin olive oil
½ sweet onion, chopped
4 cups low-sodium chicken stock
½ cup Homemade Rice Milk or unsweetened store-bought rice milk
Freshly ground black pepper
Juice of 1 lemon

Directions:

Cut the asparagus tips from the spears and set aside.

In a small stockpot over medium heat, heat the olive oil. Add the onion and cook, stirring frequently for 3 to 5 minutes, until it begins to soften.

Add the stock and asparagus stalks, and bring to a boil. Reduce the heat and simmer until the asparagus is tender, about 15 minutes.

Transfer to a blender or food processor, and carefully purée until smooth. Return to the pot, add the asparagus tips, and simmer until tender, about 5 minutes.

Add the rice milk, pepper, and lemon juice, and stir until heated through. Serve.

Cooking tip: Make this soup up to three days in advance and store in the refrigerator. When ready to serve, heat in the microwave or on the stove top.

Nutrition:

Calories: 86 | Total Fat: 11g | Cholesterol: 26mg | Carbohydrates: 17g | Fiber: 3g | Protein: 7g | Phosphorus: 155mg | Potassium: 257mg | Sodium: 128mg

CAULIFLOWER AND CHIVE SOUP

Preparation Time: 10 minutes
Cooking Time: 20 minutes
Servings: 4
Ingredients:
2 tablespoons extra-virgin olive oil
½ sweet onion, chopped
2 garlic cloves, minced
2 cups Simple Chicken Broth or low-sodium store-bought chicken stock
1 cauliflower head, broken into florets
Freshly ground black pepper
4 tablespoons (¼ cup) finely chopped chives
Directions:
In a small stockpot over medium heat, heat the olive oil. Add the onion and cook, stirring frequently, for 3 to 5 minutes, until it begins to soften. Add the garlic and stir until fragrant.
Add the broth and cauliflower, and bring to a boil. Reduce the heat and simmer until the cauliflower is tender, about 15 minutes.
Transfer the soup in batches to a blender or food processor and purée until smooth, or use an immersion blender. Return the soup to the pot, and season with pepper. Before serving, top each bowl with 1 tablespoon of chives.
Cooking tip: If you're using a traditional blender, work in batches, and place a clean kitchen towel over the top of the lid as you blend to prevent splashing hot soup. Fill the blender only to the safe-fill line, and be very cautious as you go, as hot liquids can be dangerous to work with.
Nutrition:
Calories: 156 | Total Fat: 11g | Cholesterol: 16mg | Carbohydrates: 17g | Fiber: 3g | Protein: 7g | Phosphorus: 125mg | Potassium: 527mg | Sodium: 248mg

BULGUR AND GREENS SOUP WITH SOFT-BOILED EGG

Preparation Time: 10 minutes
Cooking Time: 20 minutes
Servings: 4
Ingredients:
1 cup bulgur
4 eggs
4 cups Simple Chicken Broth or low-sodium store-bought chicken stock
1 bunch mustard greens, thick stems removed, coarsely chopped
Freshly ground black pepper
2 scallions, thinly sliced
2-inch piece ginger, julienned
2 celery stalks, thinly sliced
Directions:
In a small pot, add the bulgur to 2 cups of water and bring to a boil. Cover, reduce the heat, and simmer for 10 to 15 minutes, until the bulgur is tender. Drain the bulgur and set aside.
Place the whole eggs in a small bowl. Bring a pot of water to a boil, and carefully pour the water over the eggs. Let sit for 8 minutes, or longer if a more-set egg is desired. Carefully peel the eggs and set aside.
In a medium stockpot, bring the broth to a simmer. Add the mustard greens, season with pepper, and cook until tender, 3 to 5 minutes.
Divide the bulgur between four bowls, and add 1 cup of broth to each bowl. Divide the mustard greens between the bowls. Add 1 egg to each bowl. Top with the scallions, ginger, and celery. Serve.
Substitution tip: If you can't find mustard greens, feel free to substitute any other type of green. Turnip greens, collard greens, or spinach all work well. If you are using a green with thick stems, like turnip or collard greens, remove the stems before cooking.
Nutrition:
Calories: 86 | Total Fat: 21g | Cholesterol: 26mg | Carbohydrates: 17g | Fiber: 3g | Protein: 7g | Phosphorus: 125mg | Potassium: 537mg | Sodium: 158mg

VEGETABLE LENTIL SOUP

Preparation Time: 10 minutes
Cooking Time: 25 minutes
Servings: 4
Ingredients:
1 tablespoon extra-virgin olive oil
½ sweet onion, diced
2 carrots, diced
2 celery stalks, diced
½ cup lentils
5 cups Simple Chicken Broth or low-sodium store-bought chicken stock
2 cups sliced chard leaves
Freshly ground black pepper
Juice of 1 lemon

Directions:
In a medium stockpot over medium-high heat, heat the olive oil. Add the onion and stir until softened, about 3 to 5 minutes.
Add the carrots, celery, lentils, and broth. Bring to a boil, reduce the heat and simmer, uncovered, for 15 minutes, until the lentils are tender.
Add the chard and cook for 3 additional minutes, until wilted.
Season it with the pepper and lemon juice. Serve.
Substitution tip: You can use any greens that you have on hand for this soup; just adjust **Cooking Time**s as needed based on the type. Collard, mustard, and turnip greens will need more **Cooking Time**, while spinach or bok choy will require just a couple minutes, much like chard.
Nutrition:
Calories: 186 | Total Fat: 11g | Cholesterol: 26mg | Carbohydrates: 17g | Fiber: 3g | Protein: 7g | Phosphorus: 125mg | Potassium: 557mg | Sodium: 148mg

SIMPLE CHICKEN AND RICE SOUP

Preparation Time: 10 minutes
Cooking Time: 15 minutes
Servings: 4
Ingredients:
1 tablespoon extra-virgin olive oil
½ sweet onion, chopped
2 celery stalks, chopped
2 carrots, chopped
8 ounces chicken breast, diced
4 cups Simple Chicken Broth or low-sodium store-bought chicken stock
¼ teaspoon dried thyme leaves
1 cup cooked rice
Juice of 1 lime
Freshly ground black pepper
2 tablespoons chopped parsley leaves, for garnish

Directions:
In a medium stockpot, heat the olive oil over medium-high heat. Add the onion, celery, and carrots, and cook, stirring often, for about 5 minutes, until the onion begins to soften.
Add the chicken breast and continue stirring until the meat is just browned but not cooked through.
Add the broth and thyme, and bring to a boil.
Reduce the heat and simmer for 10 minutes, until the chicken is cooked through and the vegetables are tender.
Add the rice and lime juice. Season with pepper. Serve, garnished with parsley leaves.
Lower sodium tip: Choosing the Simple Chicken Broth over the store-bought variety will allow you better to control the amount of sodium in the finished product.
Nutrition:
Calories: 176 | Total Fat: 11g | Cholesterol: 26mg | Carbohydrates: 17g| Fiber: 3g | Protein: 7g | Phosphorus: 225mg | Potassium: 357mg | Sodium: 128mg

CHICKEN PHO	TURKEY BURGER SOUP
Preparation Time: 10 minutes *Cooking Time: 15 minutes* *Servings: 4* **Ingredients:** *5 cups Simple Chicken Broth or low-sodium store-bought chicken stock* *1-inch piece ginger, cut lengthwise into 2 or 3 strips* *1 cup cooked chicken breast, diced* *Several fresh Thai basil sprigs* *1 cup mung bean sprouts* *1 lime, cut into wedges* *1 jalapeño pepper, stemmed, seeded, and thinly sliced* *1 (16-ounce) package dried rice vermicelli noodles, cooked according to package* **Directions** *4 tablespoons (¼ cup) sliced scallions* *4 tablespoons (¼ cup) chopped cilantro leaves* **Directions:** In a medium stockpot over medium-high heat, add the broth and ginger, and bring to a simmer. Add the chicken and simmer for 5 minutes. Remove the ginger from the pot and discard. On a plate, arrange the Thai basil, bean sprouts, lime wedges, and jalapeño slices. Distribute the noodles among four bowls. Add 1¼ cups of broth to each bowl. Top with 1 tablespoon each of the scallions and cilantro. Serve immediately, alongside the plate of garnishes. Substitution tip: If you can't find fresh Thai basil near you, you can substitute regular basil, available in the fresh herb section of your grocery store. **Nutrition:** *Calories: 176	Total Fat: 31g	Cholesterol: 26mg	Carbohydrates: 17g	Fiber: 3g	Protein: 7g	Phosphorus: 225mg	Potassium: 527mg	Sodium: 138mg*	*Preparation Time: 10 minutes* *Cooking Time: 25 minutes* *Servings: 4* **Ingredients:** *2 tablespoons extra-virgin olive oil* *1-pound ground turkey breast* *½ sweet onion, chopped* *3 garlic cloves, minced* *Freshly ground black pepper* *1 (16-ounce) can low-sodium diced tomatoes, drained* *4 cups Simple Chicken Broth or low-sodium store-bought chicken stock* *1 cup sliced carrots* *1 cup sliced celery* *1 tablespoon chopped fresh basil* *1 tablespoon chopped fresh oregano* *1 tablespoon chopped fresh thyme* **Directions:** In a medium stockpot over medium-high heat, heat the olive oil. Add the turkey, onion, and garlic, and cook, stirring frequently, until the turkey is browned. Season with pepper. Add the drained tomatoes, broth, carrots, celery, basil, oregano, and thyme. Reduce the heat to low, and simmer for 20 minutes. Serve. Substitution tip: If you don't have fresh basil, oregano, or thyme, use dried instead. Substitute 1 teaspoon of dried herbs for each tablespoon of fresh. **Nutrition:** Calories: 186	Fat: 11g	Cholesterol: 26mg	Carbohydrates: 17g	Fiber: 3g	Protein: 7g	Phosphorus: 115mg	Potassium: 257mg	Sodium: 128mg

TURKEY, WILD RICE, AND MUSHROOM SOUP

Preparation Time: 15 minutes
Cooking Time: 2-3 hours
Servings: 6
Ingredients:
½ cup onion, chopped
½ cup red bell pepper, chopped
½ cup carrots, chopped
2 garlic cloves, minced
2 cup cooked turkey, shredded
5 cup chicken broth (see recipe)
½ cup quick-cooking wild rice, uncooked
1 tbsp olive oil
1 cup mushrooms, sliced
2 bay leaves
¼ tsp Mrs. Dash® Original salt-free herb seasoning blend
1 tsp dried thyme
½ tsp low sodium salt
¼ tsp black pepper
Directions:
Cook rice in a saucepan with 1-2 cups of broth. Set aside.
Heat the oil in a skillet and sauté the onion, bell pepper, carrots, and garlic until soft. Add to a 4 to 6-quart slow cooker.
Add remaining **Ingredients** to the slow cooker except for the rice and mushrooms.
Cover and cook for 2-3 hours on LOW.
Add the mushrooms and rice and cook for a further 15 minutes.
Remove the bay leaves and serve.
Nutrition:
Calories: 136 | Fat: 11g | Cholesterol: 26mg | Carbohydrates: 15g | Fiber: 3g | Protein: 5g | Phosphorus: 145mg | Potassium: 537mg | Sodium: 128mg

GREEN CHILI STEW

Preparation Time: 20 minutes
Cooking Time: 10 hours
Servings: 6
Ingredients:
½ cup all-purpose flour
1 tbsp garlic powder
1 tsp black pepper
1lb lean boneless pork chops, cut into 1-inch cubes
1 tbsp olive oil
1 8oz can of green chili peppers, drained well and chopped
1 garlic clove, minced
2 cup chicken broth (see recipe)
6 flour tortillas, burrito size
¾ cup iceberg lettuce, shredded
¼ cup cilantro, finely chopped
6 tbsp sour cream
Directions:
Place the flour, garlic powder, and black pepper into a Ziploc bag.
Add the pork and coat well.
Heat the oil in a skillet and brown the pork.
Add the pork to a 4-quart slow cooker along with the broth, peppers, and garlic.
Cover and cook for 10 hours on LOW.
Place lettuce on a tortilla, top with stew and roll up burrito style.
Top with sour cream and cilantro.
Nutrition:
Calories: 126 | Fat: 11g | Cholesterol: 26mg | Carbohydrates: 17g | Fiber: 3g | Protein: 7g | Phosphorus: 155mg | Potassium: 357mg | Sodium: 188mg

Chapter 13: Vegetables

COLLARD GREEN WRAP

Preparation Time: 10 minutes
Cooking Time: 0 minutes
Servings: 4
Ingredients:
½ block feta, cut into 4 (1-inch thick) strips (4-oz)
½ cup purple onion, diced
½ medium red bell pepper, julienned
1 medium cucumber, julienned
4 large cherry tomatoes, halved
4 large collard green leaves, washed
8 whole kalamata olives, halved
Sauce Ingredients:
1 cup low-fat plain Greek yogurt
1 tablespoon white vinegar
1 teaspoon garlic powder
2 tablespoons minced fresh dill
2 tablespoons olive oil
2.5-ounces cucumber, seeded and grated (¼-whole)
Salt and pepper to taste
Directions:
Make the sauce first: make sure to squeeze out all the excess liquid from the cucumber after grating. In a small bowl, mix all sauce ingredients thoroughly and refrigerate.
Prepare and slice all wrap ingredients.
On a flat surface, spread one collard green leaf. Spread 2 tablespoons of Tzatziki sauce on middle of the leaf. The tomatoes, feta, olives, onion, pepper, and cucumber should be layer ¼ each. Place them on the center of the leaf, like piling them high instead of spreading them.
Fold the leaf like you would a burrito. Repeat process for remaining ingredients.
Serve and enjoy.
Nutrition:
Calories 463 | Fat 31g | Carbs 31g | Protein 20g | Fiber 7g | Sodium 795mg | Potassium 960mg

ZUCCHINI GARLIC FRIES

Preparation Time: 10 minutes
Cooking Time: 20 minutes
Servings: 6
Ingredients:
¼ teaspoon garlic powder
½ cup almond flour
2 large egg whites, beaten
3 medium zucchinis, sliced into fry sticks
Salt and pepper to taste
Directions:
Preheat oven to 400oF.
Mix all ingredients in a bowl until the zucchini fries are well coated.
Place fries on cookie sheet and spread evenly.
Put in oven and cook for 20 minutes.
Halfway through **Cooking Time**, stir fries.

Nutrition:
Calories 11 | Fat 0.1g | Carbs 1g | Protein1.5 g | Fiber 0.5g | Sodium 19mg | Potassium 71mg

MASHED CAULIFLOWER	STIR-FRIED EGGPLANT
Preparation Time: 10 minutes *Cooking Time: 10 minutes* *Servings: 3* **Ingredients:** *1 cauliflower head* *1 tablespoon olive oil* *½ tsp salt* *¼ tsp dill* *Pepper to taste* *2 tbsp low fat milk* **Directions:** Bring a small pot of water to a boil. Chop cauliflower in florets. Add florets to boiling water and boil uncovered for 5 minutes. Turn off fire and let it sit for 5 minutes more. In a blender, add all ingredients except for cauliflower and blend to mix well. Drain cauliflower well and add into blender. Puree until smooth and creamy. Serve and enjoy. **Nutrition** *Calories 78 | Fat 5g | Carbs 6g | Protein 2g | Fiber 2g | Sodium 420mg | Potassium 327mg*	*Preparation Time: 10 minutes* *Cooking Time: 10 minutes* *Servings: 2* **Ingredients:** *1 tablespoon coconut oil* *2 eggplants, sliced into 3-inch in length* *4 cloves of garlic, minced* *1 onion, chopped* *1 teaspoon ginger, grated* *1 teaspoon lemon juice, freshly squeezed* *½ tsp salt* *½ tsp pepper* **Directions:** Heat the oil in a nonstick saucepan. Pan-fry the eggplants for 2 minutes on all sides. Add the garlic and onions until fragrant, around 3 minutes. Stir in the ginger, salt, pepper, and lemon juice. Add a ½ cup of water and bring to a simmer. Cook until eggplant is tender. **Nutrition** *Calories 232 | Fat 8g | Carbs 41g | Protein 7g | Fiber 18g | Sodium 596mg | Potassium 1404mg*

SAUTÉED GARLIC MUSHROOMS	STIR FRIED ASPARAGUS AND BELL PEPPER
Preparation Time: 10 minutes *Cooking Time: 10 minutes* *Servings: 4* **Ingredients:** *1 tablespoon olive oil* *3 cloves of garlic, minced* *16 ounces fresh brown mushrooms, sliced* *7 ounces fresh shiitake mushrooms, sliced* *½ tsp salt* *½ tsp pepper or more to taste* **Directions:** Place a nonstick saucepan on medium high fire and heat pan for a minute. Add oil and heat for 2 minutes. Stir in garlic and sauté for a minute. Add remaining ingredients and stir fry until soft and tender, around 5 minutes. Turn off fire, let mushrooms rest while pan is covered for 5 minutes. Serve and enjoy. **Nutrition** *Calories 95	Fat 4g	Carbs 14g	Protein 3g	Fiber 4g	Sodium 296mg	Potassium 490mg*	*Preparation Time: 10 minutes* *Cooking Time: 10 minutes* *Servings: 6* **Ingredients:** *1 tablespoon olive oil* *4 cloves of garlic, minced* *1-pound fresh asparagus spears, trimmed* *2 large red bell peppers, seeded and julienned* *½ teaspoon thyme* *5 tablespoons water* *½ tsp salt* *½ tsp pepper or more to taste* **Directions:** Place a nonstick saucepan on high fire and heat pan for a minute. Add oil and heat for 2 minutes. Stir in garlic and sauté for a minute. Add remaining ingredients and stir fry until soft and tender, around 6 minutes. Turn off fire, let veggies rest while pan is covered for 5 minutes. Serve and enjoy. **Nutrition** *Calories 45	Fat 2g	Carbs 5g	Protein 2g	Fiber 2g	Sodium 482mg	Potassium 219mg*

STIR FRIED BRUSSELS SPROUTS AND PECANS

Preparation Time: 10 minutes
Cooking Time: 10 minutes
Servings: 7
Ingredients:
1 ½ pounds fresh Brussels sprouts, trimmed and halved
1 tablespoon olive oil
4 cloves of garlic, minced
3 tablespoons water
¼ tsp salt
½ tsp pepper or more to taste
½ cup chopped pecans
Directions:
Place a nonstick saucepan on high fire and heat pan for a minute.
Add oil and heat for 2 minutes.
Stir in garlic and sauté for a minute.
Add remaining ingredients and stir fry until soft and tender, around 6 minutes.
Turn off fire, let veggies rest while pan is covered for 5 minutes.
Serve and enjoy.

Nutrition
Calories 112 | Fat 7g | Carbs 11g | Protein 4g | Sugar: 4g | Fiber 3g | Sodium 108mg | Potassium 425mg

STIR FRIED KALE

Preparation Time: 10 minutes
Cooking Time: 10 minutes
Servings: 6
Ingredients:
1 tablespoon coconut oil
2 cloves of garlic, minced
1 onion, chopped
2 teaspoons crushed red pepper flakes
4 cups kale, chopped
2 tbsp water
Salt and pepper to taste
Directions:
Place a nonstick saucepan on high fire and heat pan for a minute.
Add oil and heat for 2 minutes.
Stir in garlic and sauté for a minute. Add onions and stir fry for another minute.
Add remaining ingredients and stir fry until soft and tender, around 4 minutes.
Turn off fire, let veggies rest while pan is covered for 3 minutes.
Serve and enjoy.

Nutrition
Calories 37 | Fat 2g | Carbs 4g | Protein 1g | Fiber 1g | Sodium 6mg | Potassium 111mg

STIR FRIED BOK CHOY	VEGETABLE CURRY
Preparation Time: 10 minutes *Cooking Time: 12 minutes* *Servings: 1* **Ingredients:** *1 tablespoon coconut oil* *4 cloves of garlic, minced* *1 onion, chopped* *2 heads bok choy, rinsed and chopped* *¼ tsp salt* *½ tsp pepper or more to taste* *1 tablespoons sesame seeds* **Directions:** Place a nonstick saucepan on high fire and heat pan for a minute. Add sesame seeds and toast for a minute. Transfer to a bowl. In same pan, add oil and heat for 2 minutes. Stir in garlic and sauté for a minute. Add onions and stir fry for another minute. Add remaining ingredients and stir fry until soft and tender, around 4 minutes. Turn off fire, let veggies rest while pan is covered for 3 minutes. Serve and enjoy. **Nutrition** *Calories 334 | Fat 20g | Carbs 36g | Protein 12g | Fiber 14g | Sodium 731mg | Potassium 1043mg*	*Preparation Time: 10 minutes* *Cooking Time: 20 minutes* *Servings: 4* **Ingredients:** *1 tablespoon coconut oil* *1 medium onion, chopped* *1 teaspoon minced garlic* *1 teaspoon minced ginger* *2 cup broccoli florets* *2 cups fresh spinach leaves* *1 tablespoon garam masala* *½ cup coconut milk* *½ tsp salt* *½ tsp pepper* **Directions:** Place a nonstick pot on high fire and heat pot for a minute. Add oil and heat for 2 minutes. Stir in garlic and ginger, sauté for a minute. Add onions and garam masala and stir fry for another minute. Add remaining ingredients, except for spinach leaves and simmer for 10 minutes. Stir in spinach leaves, turn off fire, let veggies rest while pot is covered for 5 minutes. Serve and enjoy. **Nutrition** *Calories 121 | Fat 11g | Carbs 6g | Protein 2g | Fiber 2g | Sodium 315mg | Potassium 266mg*

BRAISED CARROTS 'N KALE

Preparation Time: 10 minutes
Cooking Time: 10 minutes
Servings: 2
Ingredients:
1 tablespoon coconut oil
1 onion, sliced thinly
5 cloves of garlic, minced
3 medium carrots, sliced thinly
10 ounces of kale, chopped
½ cup water
Salt and pepper to taste
A dash of red pepper flakes
Directions:
Heat the oil in a skillet over medium flame and sauté the onion and garlic until fragrant.
Toss in the carrots and stir for 1 minute. Add the kale and water. Season it with salt and pepper to taste.
Close the lid and allow simmering for 5 minutes.
Sprinkle with red pepper flakes.
Serve and enjoy.
Nutrition
Calories 161 | Fat 8g | Carbs 20g | Protein 8g | Fiber 6g | Sodium 63mg | Potassium 900mg

BUTTERNUT SQUASH HUMMUS

Preparation Time: 10 minutes
Cooking Time: 15 minutes
Servings: 8
Ingredients:
2 pounds butternut squash, seeded and peeled
1 tablespoon olive oil
¼ cup tahini
2 tablespoons lemon juice
2 cloves of garlic, minced
Salt and pepper to taste
Directions:
Heat the oven to 3000F.
Coat the butternut squash with olive oil.
Place in a baking dish and bake for 15 minutes in the oven.
Once the squash is cooked, place in a food processor together with the rest of the ingredients.
Pulse it until smooth.
Place in individual containers.
Put a label and store in the fridge.
Allow to warm at room temperature before heating in the microwave oven.
Serve with carrots or celery sticks.
Nutrition
Calories 109 | Fat 6g | Carbs 15g | Protein 2g | Fiber 4g | Sodium 14mg | Potassium 379mg

STIR FRIED GINGERY VEGGIES

Preparation Time: 10 minutes
Cooking Time: 10 minutes
Servings: 4
Ingredients:
1 tablespoon oil
3 cloves of garlic, minced
1 onion, chopped
1 thumb-size ginger, sliced
1 tablespoon water
1 large carrot, peeled and julienned
1 large green bell pepper, seeded and julienned
1 large yellow bell pepper, seeded and julienned
1 large red bell pepper, seeded and julienned
1 zucchini, julienned
Salt and pepper to taste
Directions:
Heat oil in a nonstick saucepan over high flame and sauté the garlic, onion, and ginger until fragrant.
Stir in the rest of the ingredients.
Keep on stirring for at least 5 minutes until vegetables are tender.
Serve and enjoy.
Nutrition
Calories 70 | Fat 4g | Carbs 9g | Protein 1g | Fiber 2g | Sodium 273mg | Potassium 263mg | Vegetables 2

CAULIFLOWER FRITTERS

Preparation Time: 10 minutes
Cooking Time: 15 minutes
Servings: 6
Ingredients:
1 large cauliflower head, cut into florets
2 eggs, beaten
½ teaspoon turmeric
½ teaspoon salt
¼ teaspoon black pepper
1 tablespoon coconut oil
Directions:
Place the cauliflower florets in a pot with water and bring to a boil. Cook until tender, around 5 minutes of boiling. Drain well.
Place the cauliflower, eggs, turmeric, salt, and pepper into the food processor.
Pulse until the mixture becomes coarse.
Transfer into a bowl. Using your hands, form six small flattened balls and place in the fridge for at least 1 hour until the mixture hardens.
Heat the oil in a nonstick pan and fry the cauliflower patties for 3 minutes on each side.
Serve and enjoy.

Nutrition
Calories 53 | Fat 6g | Carbs 2g | Protein 3g | Fiber 1g | Sodium 228mg | Potassium 159mg

STIR-FRIED SQUASH

Preparation Time: 10 minutes
Cooking Time: 10 minutes
Servings: 4
Ingredients:
1 tablespoon olive oil
3 cloves of garlic, minced
1 butternut squash, seeded and sliced
1 tablespoon coconut aminos
1 tablespoon lemon juice
1 tablespoon water
Salt and pepper to taste
Directions:
Heat the oil over medium flame and sauté the garlic until fragrant.

Stir in the squash for another 3 minutes before adding the rest of the ingredients.

Close the lid and allow to simmer for 5 more minutes or until the squash is soft.

Serve and enjoy.
Nutrition
Calories 83 | Fat 3g | Carbs 14g | Protein 2g | Fiber 2g | Sodium 8mg | Potassium 211mg

Chapter 14: Seafood

CURRIED FISH CAKES

Preparation time: 10 minutes
Cooking time: 18 minutes
Servings: 4
Ingredients
¾ pound atlantic cod, cubed
1 apple, peeled and cubed
1 tablespoon yellow curry paste
2 tablespoons cornstarch
1 tablespoon peeled grated ginger root
1 large egg
1 tablespoon freshly squeezed lemon juice
⅛ teaspoon freshly ground black pepper
½ cup crushed puffed rice cereal
1 tablespoon olive oil

Directions
Put the cod, apple, curry, cornstarch, ginger, egg, lemon juice, and pepper in a blender or food processor and process until finely chopped. Avoid over-processing, or the mixture will become mushy.
Place the rice cereal on a shallow plate.
Form the mixture into 8 patties.
Dredge the patties in the rice cereal to coat.
Cook patties for 3 to 5 minutes per side, turning once until a meat thermometer registers 160°f.
Serve.
Nutrition:
Calories: 188 | Total fat: 6g | Saturated fat: 1g | Sodium: 150mg | Potassium: 292mg| Phosphorus: 150mg | Carbohydrates: 12g | Fiber: 1g | Protein: 21g | Sugar: 5g

BAKED SOLE WITH CARAMELIZED ONION

Preparation time: 10 minutes
Cooking time: 20 minutes
Servings: 4
Ingredients
1 cup finely chopped onion
½ cup low-sodium vegetable broth
1 yellow summer squash, sliced
2 cups frozen broccoli florets
4 (3-ounce) fillets of sole
Pinch salt
2 tablespoons olive oil
Pinch baking soda
2 teaspoons avocado oil
1 teaspoon dried basil leaves

Directions
Preheat the oven to 425°f.
Add the onions. Cook for 1 minute; then, stirring constantly, cook for another 4 minutes.
Remove the onions from the heat.
Pour the broth into a baking sheet with a lip and arrange the squash and broccoli on the sheet in a single layer. Top the vegetables with the fish. Sprinkle the fish with the salt and drizzle everything with the olive oil.
Bake the fish and the vegetables for 10 minutes.
While the fish is baking, return the skillet with the onions to medium-high heat and stir in a pinch of baking soda. Stir in the avocado oil and cook for 5 minutes, stirring frequently, until the onions are dark brown.
Transfer the onions to a plate.
Tp the fish evenly with the onions. Sprinkle with the basil.
Return the fish to the oven, after this bake it 8 to10 minutes serve the fish on the vegetables.
Nutrition:
Calories: 202 | Total fat: 11g | Saturated fat: 3g | Sodium: 320mg | Potassium: 537 |Phosphorus: 331mg | Carbohydrates: 10g | Fiber: 3g | Protein: 16g | Sugar: 4g

THAI TUNA WRAPS

Preparation time: 10 minutes
Cooking time: 0 minute
Servings: 4
Ingredients
¼ cup unsalted peanut butter
2 tablespoons freshly squeezed lemon juice
1 teaspoon low-sodium soy sauce
½ teaspoon ground ginger
⅛ teaspoon cayenne pepper
1 (6-ounce) can no-salt-added or low-sodium chunk light tuna, drained
1 cup shredded red cabbage
2 scallions, white and green parts, chopped
1 cup grated carrots
8 butter lettuce leaves

Directions
In a medium bowl, stir together the peanut butter, lemon juice, soy sauce, ginger, and cayenne pepper until well combined.
Stir in the tuna, cabbage, scallions, and carrots.
Divide the tuna filling evenly between the butter lettuce leaves and serve.
Nutrition:
Calories: 175 | Total fat; 10g | Saturated fat: 1g | Sodium: 98mg | Potassium: 421mg | Phosphorus: 153mg | Carbohydrates: 8g | Fiber: 2g | Protein: 17g | Sugar: 4g

GRILLED FISH AND VEGETABLE PACKETS

Preparation time: 15 minutes
Cooking time: 12 minutes
Servings: 4
Ingredients
1 (8-ounce) package sliced mushrooms
1 leek, white and green parts, chopped
1 cup frozen corn
4 (4-ounce) atlantic cod fillets
Juice of 1 lemon
3 tablespoons olive oil
Directions
Prepare and preheat the grill to medium coals and set a grill 6 inches from the coals.
Tear off four 30-inch long strips of heavy-duty aluminum foil.
Arrange the mushrooms, leek, and corn in the center of each piece of foil and top with the fish.
Drizzle the packet contents evenly with the lemon juice and olive oil.
Bring the longer length sides of the foil together at the top and, holding the edges together, fold them over twice and then fold in the width sides to form a sealed packet with room for the steam.
Put the packets on the grill and grill for 10 to 12 minutes until the vegetables are tender-crisp and the fish flakes when tested with a fork. Be careful opening the packets because the escaping steam can be scalding.
Nutrition:
Calories: 267 | Total fat: 12g | Saturated fat: 2g | Sodium: 97mg | Potassium: 582mg | Phosphorus: 238mg | Carbohydrates: 13g | Fiber: 2g | Protein: 29g | Sugar: 3g

WHITE FISH SOUP	LEMON BUTTER SALMON
Preparation time: 15 minutes *Cooking time: 20 minutes* *Servings: 4* **Ingredients** 2 tablespoons olive oil 1 onion, finely diced 1 green bell pepper, chopped 1 rib celery, thinly sliced 3 cups chicken broth, or more to taste 1/4 cup chopped fresh parsley 1 1/2 pounds cod, cut into 3/4-inch cubes Pepper to taste 1 dash red pepper flakes **Directions** Heat oil in a soup pot over medium heat. Add onion, bell pepper, and celery and cook until wilted, about 5 minutes. Add broth and then bring to a simmer, about 5 minutes. Cook 15 to 20 minutes. Add cod, parsley, and red pepper flakes and simmer until fish flakes easily with a fork, 8 to 10 minutes more. Season with black pepper. **Nutrition:** *Calories 117 | Total fat 7.2g | Saturated fat 1.4g | Cholesterol 18mg | Sodium 37mg | Total carbohydrate 5.4g | Dietary fiber 1.3g | Total sugars 2.8g | Protein 8.1g | Calcium 23mg | Iron 1mg | Potassium 122mg | Phosphorus 111 mg*	*Preparation time: 15 minutes* *Cooking time: 15 minutes* *Servings: 6* **Ingredients** *1 tablespoon butter* *2 tablespoons olive oil* *1 tablespoon dijon mustard* *1 tablespoons lemon juice* *2 cloves garlic, crushed* *1 teaspoon dried dill* *1 teaspoon dried basil leaves* *1 tablespoon capers* *24-ounce salmon filet* **Directions** Put all of the ingredients except the salmon in a saucepan over medium heat. Bring to a boil and then simmer for 5 minutes. Preheat your grill. Create a packet using foil. Place the sauce and salmon inside. Seal the packet. Grill for 12 minutes. **Nutrition:** *Calories 292 | Protein 22 g | Carbohydrates 2 g | Fat 22 g | Cholesterol 68 mg | Sodium 190 mg | Potassium 439 mg | Phosphorus 280 mg | Calcium 21 mg*

CRAB CAKE	BAKED FISH IN CREAM SAUCE
Preparation time: 15 minutes *Cooking time: 9 minutes* *Servings: 6* **Ingredients** *1/4 cup onion, chopped* *1/4 cup bell pepper, chopped* *1 egg, beaten* *6 low-sodium crackers, crushed* *1/4 cup low-fat mayonnaise* *1-pound crab meat* *1 tablespoon dry mustard* *Pepper to taste* *2 tablespoons lemon juice* *1 tablespoon fresh parsley* *1 tablespoon garlic powder* *3 tablespoons olive oil* **Directions** Mix all the ingredients except the oil. Form 6 patties from the mixture. Pour the oil into a pan in a medium heat. Cook the crab cakes for 5 minutes. Flip and cook for another 4 minutes. **Nutrition:** *Calories 189 | Protein 13 g | Carbohydrates 5 g | Fat 14 g | Cholesterol 111 mg | Sodium 342 mg | Potassium 317 mg | Phosphorus 185 mg | Calcium 52 mg | Fiber 0.5 g*	*Preparation time: 10 minutes* *Cooking time: 40 minutes* *Servings: 4* **Ingredients** *1-pound haddock* *1/2 cup all-purpose flour* *2 tablespoons butter (unsalted)* *1/4 teaspoon pepper* *2 cups fat-free nondairy creamer* *1/4 cup water* **Directions** Preheat your oven to 350 degrees f. Spray baking pan with oil. Sprinkle with a little flour. Arrange fish on the pan Season with pepper. Sprinkle remaining flour on the fish. Spread creamer on both sides of the fish. Bake for 40 minutes or until golden. Spread cream sauce on top of the fish before serving. **Nutrition:** *Calories 383 | Protein 24 g | Carbohydrates 46 g | Fat 11 g | Cholesterol 79 mg | Sodium 253 mg | Potassium 400 mg | Phosphorus 266 mg | Calcium 46 mg | Fiber 0.4 g*

SHRIMP & BROCCOLI

Preparation time: 10 minutes
Cooking time: 5 minutes
Servings: 4
Ingredients
1 tablespoon olive oil
1 clove garlic, minced
1-pound shrimp
1/4 cup red bell pepper
1 cup broccoli florets, steamed
10-ounce cream cheese
1/2 teaspoon garlic powder
1/4 cup lemon juice
3/4 teaspoon ground peppercorns
1/4 cup half and half creamer

Directions
Pour the oil and cook garlic for 30 seconds.
Add shrimp and cook for 2 minutes.
Add the rest of the ingredients.
Mix well.
Cook for 2 minutes.
Nutrition:
Calories 469 | Protein 28 g | Carbohydrates 28 g | Fat 28 g | Cholesterol 213 mg | Sodium 374 mg | Potassium 469 mg | Phosphorus 335 mg | Calcium 157 mg | Fiber 2.6 g

SHRIMP IN GARLIC SAUCE

Preparation time: 10 minutes
Cooking time: 6 minutes
Servings: 4
Ingredients
3 tablespoons butter (unsalted)
1/4 cup onion, minced
3 cloves garlic, minced
1-pound shrimp, shelled and deveined
1/2 cup half and half creamer
1/4 cup white wine
2 tablespoons fresh basil
Black pepper to taste
Directions
Add butter to a pan over medium low heat.
Let it melt.
Add the onion and garlic.
Cook for it 1-2 minutes.
Add the shrimp and cook for 2 minutes.
Transfer shrimp on a serving platter and set aside.
Add the rest of the ingredients.
Simmer for 3 minutes.
Pour sauce over the shrimp and serve.
Nutrition:
Calories 482 | Protein 33 g | Carbohydrates 46 g | Fat 11 g | Cholesterol 230 mg | Sodium 213 mg | Potassium 514 mg | Phosphorus 398 mg | Calcium 133 mg | Fiber 2.0 g

FISH TACO

Preparation time: 40 minutes
Cooking time: 10 minutes
Servings: 6
Ingredients
1 tablespoon lime juice
1 tablespoon olive oil
1 clove garlic, minced
1-pound cod fillets
1/2 teaspoon ground cumin
1/4 teaspoon black pepper
1/2 teaspoon chili powder
1/4 cup sour cream
1/2 cup mayonnaise
2 tablespoons nondairy milk
1 cup cabbage, shredded
1/2 cup onion, chopped
1/2 bunch cilantro, chopped
12 corn tortillas
Directions
Drizzle lemon juice over the fish fillet.
And then coat it with olive oil and then season with garlic, cumin, pepper and chili powder.
Let it sit for 30 minutes.
Broil fish for 10 minutes, flipping halfway through.
Flake the fish using a fork.
In a bowl, mix sour cream, milk and mayo.
Assemble tacos by filling each tortilla with mayo mixture, cabbage, onion, cilantro and fish flakes.
Nutrition:
Calories 366 | Protein 18 g | Carbohydrates 31 g | Fat 19 g | Cholesterol 40 mg | Sodium 194 mg | Potassium 507 mg | Phosphorus 327 mg | Calcium 138 mg | Fiber 4.3 g

BAKED TROUT

Preparation time: 5 minutes
Cooking time: 10 minutes
Servings: 8
Ingredients
2-pound trout fillet
1 tablespoon oil
1 teaspoon salt-free lemon pepper
1/2 teaspoon paprika
Directions
Preheat your oven to 350 **degrees** f.
Coat fillet with oil.
Place fish on a baking pan.
Season with lemon pepper and paprika.
Bake for 10 minutes.

Nutrition:
Calories 161 | Protein 21 g | Carbohydrates 0 g | Fat 8 g | Cholesterol 58 mg | Sodium 109 mg | Potassium 385 mg | Phosphorus 227 mg | Calcium 75 mg | Fiber 0.1 g

FISH WITH MUSHROOMS	SALMON WITH SPICY HONEY
Preparation time: 5 minutes *Cooking time: 16 minutes* *Servings: 4* **Ingredients** *1-pound cod fillet* *2 tablespoons butter* *¼ cup white onion, chopped* *1 cup fresh mushrooms* *1 teaspoon dried thyme* **Directions** Put the fish in a baking pan. Preheat your oven to 450 degrees f. Melt the butter and cook onion and mushroom for 1 minute. Spread mushroom mixture on top of the fish. Season with thyme. Bake in the oven for 15 minutes. **Nutrition:** *Calories 156	Protein 21 g	Carbohydrates 3 g	Fat 7 g	Cholesterol 49 mg	Sodium 110 mg	Potassium 561 mg	Phosphorus 225 mg	Calcium 30 mg	Fiber 0.5 g*	*Preparation time: 15 minutes* *Cooking time: 8 minutes* *Servings: 2* **Ingredients** *16-ounce salmon fillet* *3 tablespoon honey* *3/4 teaspoon lemon peel* *3 bowls arugula salad* *1/2 teaspoon black pepper* *1/2 teaspoon garlic powder* *2 teaspoon olive oil* *1 teaspoon hot water* **Directions** Prepare a small bowl with some hot water and put in honey, grated lemon peel, ground pepper, and garlic powder. Spread the mixture over salmon fillets. Warm some olive oil at a medium heat and add spiced salmon fillet and cook for 4 minutes. Turn the fillets on one side then on the other side. Continue to cook for other 4 minutes at a reduced heat and try to check when the salmon fillets flake easily. Put some arugula on each plate and add the salmon fillets on top, adding some aromatic herbs or some dill. Serve and enjoy! **Nutrition:** *Calories 320	Protein 23 g	Potassium 450 mg	Phosphorus 250 mg*

SALMON WITH MAPLE GLAZE

Preparation time: 15 minutes
Cooking time: 2 hours
Servings: 4

Ingredients

1-pound salmon fillets
1 tablespoon green onion, chopped
1 tablespoon low sodium soy sauce
2 garlic cloves, pressed
2 tablespoon fresh cilantro
3 tablespoon lemon juice (or juice of 1 lemon)
3 tablespoon maple syrup

Directions

Combine all ingredients except for salmon.
Put salmon on platter and then pour marinade over fillets. Let it marinate 2 hours or more.
Preheat broiler.
Remove salmon from marinade.
Place salmon on bottom rack and broil for 10 minutes. Do not turn over.
Serve hot/cold with a wedge of lemon.

Nutrition:

Calories 220 | Protein 24 g | Carbohydrates 12 g | Fat 8 g | Sodium 621 mg | Potassium 440 mg | Phosphorus 374 mg

Chapter 15: Seafood 2

STEAMED SPICY TILAPIA FILLET

Preparation Time: 10 minutes
Cooking Time: 25 minutes
Servings: 4
Ingredients
4 fillets of tilapia
1 teaspoon hot pepper sauce
1 large sprig thyme
1 tablespoon ketchup
1 tablespoon lime juice
1 cup hot water
1/2 cup onion, sliced
1/4 teaspoon black pepper
3/4 cup red and green peppers, sliced

Directions
In a large shallow dish that fits your steamer, mix well hot pepper sauce, thyme, ketchup, lemon juice, and black pepper. Mix thoroughly.
Add tilapia fillets and spoon over sauce.
Mix in remaining ingredients except for water. Mix well in sauce.
Cover top of dish with foil.
Add the hot water in the steamer. Place dish on steamer rack. Cover pot and steam fish and veggies for 20 minutes.
Let it stand for 5-6 minutes before serving.
Nutrition:
Calories per serving: 131 | Protein 24 g | Carbohydrates 5 g | Fat 3 g | Sodium 102 mg | Potassium 457 mg | Phosphorus 212 mg |

DIJON MUSTARD AND LIME MARINATED SHRIMP

Preparation time: 20 minutes
Cooking time: 80 minutes
Servings: 8
Ingredients
1-pound uncooked shrimp, peeled and deveined
1 bay leaf
3 whole cloves
½ cup rice vinegar
1 cup water
½ teaspoon hot sauce
2 tablespoons. Capers
2 tablespoons. Dijon mustard
½ cup fresh lime juice, plus lime zest as garnish
1 medium red onion, chopped

Directions
Mix hot sauce, mustard, capers, lime juice and onion in a shallow baking dish and set aside.
Bring it to a boil in a large saucepan bay leaf, cloves, vinegar and water.
Once boiling, add shrimps and cook for a minute while stirring continuously.
Drain shrimps and pour shrimps into onion mixture.
For an hour, refrigerate while covered the shrimps. Then serve shrimps cold and garnished with lime zest.
Nutrition:
Calories per serving: 123 | Protein 12 g | Carbohydrates 3 g | Fat 1 g | Sodium 568 mg | Potassium 87 mg | Phosphorus 87 mg |

BAKED COD CRUSTED WITH HERBS	DILL RELISH ON WHITE SEA BASS
Preparation time: 15 minutes *Cooking time: 10 minutes* *Servings: 4* **Ingredients** *¼ cup honey* *½ cup panko* *½ teaspoon pepper* *1 tablespoon extra-virgin olive oil* *1 tablespoon lemon juice* *1 teaspoon dried basil* *1 teaspoon dried parsley* *1 teaspoon rosemary* *4 pieces of 4-ounce cod fillets* **Directions** With olive oil, grease a 9 x 13-inch baking pan and preheat oven to 375of. In a zip top bag mix panko, rosemary, pepper, parsley and basil. Evenly spread cod fillets in prepped dish and drizzle with lemon juice. Then brush the fillets with honey on all sides. Discard remaining honey if any. Then evenly divide the panko mixture on top of cod fillets. Pop in the oven and bake for ten minutes or until fish is cooked. Serve and enjoy. **Nutrition:** *Calories per serving: 113 | Protein 5 g |* *Carbohydrates 21 g | Fat 2 g | Sodium 139 mg |* *Potassium 115 mg | Phosphorus 89 mg |*	*Preparation time: 15 minutes* *Cooking time: 60 minutes* *Servings: 4* **Ingredients** *1 lemon, quartered* *4 pieces of 4-ounce white sea bass fillets* *1 teaspoon lemon juice* *1 teaspoon dijon mustard* *1 ½ teaspoons. Chopped fresh dill* *1 teaspoon pickled baby capers, drained* *1 ½ tablespoons. Chopped white onion* **Directions** Preheat oven to 375of. Mix lemon juice, mustard, dill, capers and onions in a small bowl. Prepare four aluminum foil squares and place 1 fillet per foil. Squeeze a lemon wedge per fish. Evenly divide into 4 the dill spread and drizzle over fillet. Close the foil over the fish securely and pop in the oven. Bake for 9 to 12 minutes or until fish is cooked through. Remove from foil and transfer to a serving platter, serve and enjoy. **Nutrition:** *Calories per serving: 71 | Protein 7 g |* *Carbohydrates 11 g | Fat 7 g | Sodium 94 mg |* *Potassium 237 mg | Phosphorus 91 mg |*

TILAPIA WITH LEMON GARLIC SAUCE

Preparation time: 15 minutes
Cooking time: 30 minutes
Servings: 4
Ingredients
Pepper
1 teaspoon dried parsley flakes
1 clove garlic (finely chopped)
1 tablespoon butter (melted)
3 tablespoons. Fresh lemon juice
4 tilapia fillets
Directions
First, spray baking dish with non-stick cooking spray then preheat oven at 375 degrees fahrenheit (190oc).
In cool water, rinse tilapia fillets and using paper towels pat dry the fillets.
Place tilapia fillets in the baking dish then pour butter and lemon juice and top off with pepper, parsley and garlic.
Bake tilapia in the preheated oven for 30 minutes and wait until fish is white.
Enjoy!
Nutrition:
Calories per serving: 168 | Protein 24 g | Carbohydrates 4 g | Fat 5 g | Sodium 85 mg | Potassium 431 mg | Phosphorus 207 mg |

SPINACH WITH TUSCAN WHITE BEANS AND SHRIMPS

Preparation time: 5 minutes
Cooking time: 15 minutes
Servings: 4
Ingredients
1 ½ ounces crumbled reduce-fat feta cheese
5 cups baby spinach
15 ounces can no salt added cannellini beans (rinsed and drained)
½ cup low sodium, fat-free chicken broth
2 tablespoons. Balsamic vinegar
2 teaspoons. Chopped fresh sage
4 cloves garlic (minced)
1 medium onion (chopped)
1-pound large shrimp (peeled and deveined)
2 tablespoons. Olive oil

Directions
Heat 1 teaspoon oil. Heat it over medium-high. Then for about 2 to 3 minutes, cook the shrimps using the heated skillet then place them on a plate. Heat on the same skillet the sage, garlic, and onions then cook for about 4 minutes. Add and stir in vinegar for 30 seconds.
For about 2 minutes, add chicken broth. Then, add spinach and beans and cook for an additional 2 to 3 minutes.
Remove skillet then add and stir in cooked shrimps topped with feta cheese.
Serve and divide into 4 bowls. Enjoy!
Nutrition:
Calories per serving: 343 | Protein 22 g | Carbohydrates 21 g | Fat 11 g | Sodium 766 mg | Potassium 599 mg | Phosphorus 400 mg |

BAGEL WITH SALMON AND EGG

Preparation time: 15 minutes
Cooking time: 10 minutes
Servings: 1
Ingredients
Bagel – ½
Cream cheese – 1 tablespoon
Scallions – 1 tablespoon
Fresh dill – ½ teaspoon
Fresh basil leaves – 2
Tomato – 1 slice
Arugula – 4 pieces
Egg – 1 large
Cooked salmon – 1 ounce

Directions
Start by slicing the bagel through the center horizontally. Take one half of the bagel and toast it in an oven or a toaster.
Finely chop the dill, basil leaves, and scallions. Set aside.
Add in the cream cheese. Toss in the chopped dill, basil, and scallions. Mix well to combine. Take the toasted bagel and spread the herbs and cream cheese mixture evenly over it.
Place the tomato slice and arugula on top. Set aside.
Take a small mixing bowl and then beat the egg.
Take a non-stick saucepan and grease it using cooking spray. Stir after pouring the beaten egg into the pan and. Cook for about 1 minute over medium heat. Keep stirring to make a perfect scrambled egg.
Take the cooked salmon and place it in the same pan as the egg. This will help you heat the salmon and cook the egg at the same time.
Place the scrambled egg over the tomato slice and top it with the salmon.
Nutrition:
Carbohydrates 29 g | Fat 14 g | Sodium 378 mg | Potassium 338 mg | Phosphorus 270 mg |Cholesterol 218 mg | Fiber 2.6 g |Calcium 77m

SALMON STUFFED PASTA

Preparation time: 20 minutes
Cooking time: 35 minutes
Servings: 24
Ingredients:
24 jumbo pasta shells, boiled
1 cup coffee creamer
Filling:
2 eggs, beaten
2 cups creamed cottage cheese
¼ cup chopped onion
1 red bell pepper, diced
2 teaspoons dried parsley
½ teaspoon lemon peel
1 can salmon, drained
Dill Sauce:
1 ½ teaspoon butter
1 ½ teaspoon flour
1/8 teaspoon pepper
1 tablespoon lemon juice
1 ½ cup coffee creamer
2 teaspoons dried dill weed
Direction:
Beat the cream cheese with the egg and all the other filling ingredients in a bowl.
Divide the filling in the pasta shells and place the shells in a 9x13 baking dish.
Pour the coffee creamer around the stuffed shells then cover with a foil.
Bake the shells for 30 minutes at 350 degrees F.
Meanwhile, whisk all the ingredients for dill sauce in a saucepan.
Stir for 5 minutes until it thickens.
Pour this sauce over the baked pasta shells.
Serve warm.
Nutrition:
Calories 268 | Total Fat 4.8g | Sodium 86mg | Protein 11.5g | Calcium 27mg | Phosphorous 314mg | Potassium 181mg

HERBED VEGETABLE TROUT

Preparation time: 15 minutes
Cooking time: 15 minutes
Servings: 4
Ingredients:
14 oz. trout fillets
1/2 teaspoon herb seasoning blend
1 lemon, sliced
2 green onions, sliced
1 stalk celery, chopped
1 medium carrot, julienne
Direction:
Prepare and preheat a charcoal grill over moderate heat.
Place the trout fillets over a large piece of foil and drizzle herb seasoning on top.
Spread the lemon slices, carrots, celery, and green onions over the fish.
Cover the fish with foil and pack it.
Place the packed fish in the grill and cook for 15 minutes.
Once done, remove the foil from the fish.
Serve.
Nutrition:
Calories 202 | Total Fat 8.5g | Sodium 82mg | Calcium 70mg | Phosphorous 287mg | Potassium 560mg

CITRUS GLAZED SALMON

Preparation time: 20 minutes
Cooking time: 17 minutes
Servings: 4
Ingredients:
2 garlic cloves, crushed
1 1/2 tablespoons lemon juice
2 tablespoons olive oil
1 tablespoon butter
1 tablespoon Dijon mustard
2 dashes cayenne pepper
1 teaspoon dried basil leaves
1 teaspoon dried dill
24 oz. salmon filet

Direction:
Place a 1-quart saucepan over moderate heat and add the oil, butter, garlic, lemon juice, mustard, cayenne pepper, dill, and basil to the pan.
Stir this mixture for 5 minutes after it has boiled.
Prepare and preheat a charcoal grill over moderate heat.
Place the fish on a foil sheet and fold the edges to make a foil tray.
Pour the prepared sauce over the fish.
Place the fish in the foil in the preheated grill and cook for 12 minutes.
Slice and serve.
Nutrition:
Calories 401 | Total Fat 20.5g | Cholesterol 144mg | Sodium 256mg | Carbohydrate 0.5g | Calcium 549mg | Phosphorous 214mg | Potassium 446mg

BROILED SALMON FILLETS

Preparation time: 10 minutes
Cooking time: 13 minutes
Servings: 4
Ingredients:
1 tablespoon ginger root, grated
1 clove garlic, minced
¼ cup maple syrup
1 tablespoon hot pepper sauce
4 salmon fillets, skinless
Direction:
Grease a pan with cooking spray and place it over moderate heat.
Add the ginger and garlic and sauté for 3 minutes then transfer to a bowl.
Add the hot pepper sauce and maple syrup to the ginger-garlic.
Mix well and keep this mixture aside.
Place the salmon fillet in a suitable baking tray, greased with cooking oil.
Brush the maple sauce over the fillets liberally
Broil them for 10 minutes at the oven at broiler settings.
Serve warm.
Nutrition:
Calories 289 | Total Fat 11.1g | Sodium 80mg | Carbohydrate 13.6g | Calcium 78mg | Phosphorous 230mg | Potassium 331mg

BROILED SHRIMP

Preparation time: 10 minutes
Cooking time: 5 minutes
Servings: 8
Ingredients:
1 lb. shrimp in shell
1/2 cup unsalted butter, melted
2 teaspoons lemon juice
2 tablespoons chopped onion
1 clove garlic, minced
1/8 teaspoon pepper
Direction:
Toss the shrimp with the butter, lemon juice, onion, garlic, and pepper in a bowl.
Spread the seasoned shrimp in a baking tray.
Broil for 5 minutes in an oven on broiler setting.
Serve warm.

Nutrition:
Calories 164 | Total Fat 12.8g | Sodium 242mg | Carbohydrate 0.6g | Calcium 45mg | Phosphorous 215mg | Potassium 228mg

GRILLED LEMONY COD	SPICED HONEY SALMON
Preparation time: 10 minutes *Cooking time: 10 minutes* *Servings: 4* **Ingredients:** *1 lb. cod fillets* *1 teaspoon salt-free lemon pepper seasoning* *1/4 cup lemon juice* **Direction:** Rub the cod fillets with lemon pepper seasoning and lemon juice. Grease a baking tray with cooking spray and place the salmon in the baking tray. Bake the fish for 10 minutes at 350 degrees F in a preheated oven. Serve warm. **Nutrition:** *Calories 155 | Total Fat 7.1g | Cholesterol 50mg | Sodium 53mg | Protein 22.2g | Calcium 43mg | Phosphorous 237mg | Potassium 461mg*	*Preparation time: 15 minutes* *Cooking time: 16 minutes* *Servings: 4* **Ingredients:** *3 tablespoons honey* *3/4 teaspoon lemon peel* *1/2 teaspoon black pepper* *1/2 teaspoon garlic powder* *1 teaspoon water* *16 oz. salmon fillets* *2 tablespoons olive oil* *Dill, chopped, to serve* **Direction:** Whisk the lemon peel with honey, garlic powder, hot water, and ground pepper in a small bowl. Rub this honey mixture over the salmon fillet liberally. Set a suitable skillet over moderate heat and add olive oil to heat. Set the spiced salmon fillets in the pan and sear them for 4 minutes per side. Garnish with dill. Serve warm. **Nutrition:** *Calories 264 | Total Fat 14.1g | Cholesterol 50mg | Sodium 55mg | Calcium 67mg | Phosphorous 174mg | Potassium 507mg*

Chapter 16: Poultry

GROUND CHICKEN WITH BASIL

Preparation time: fifteen minutes
Cooking time: 16 minutes
Servings: 8
Ingredients
2 pounds lean ground chicken
3 tablespoons coconut oil, divided
1 zucchini, chopped
1 red bell pepper, seeded and chopped
½ of green bell pepper, seeded and chopped
4 garlic cloves, minced
1 (1-inch) piece fresh ginger, minced
1 (1-inch) piece fresh turmeric, minced
1 fresh red chile, sliced thinly
1 tablespoon organic honey
1 tablespoon coconut amino
1½ tablespoons fish sauce
½ cup fresh basil, chopped
Salt and freshly ground black pepper, to taste
1 tablespoon fresh lime juice
Directions
Heat a large skillet on medium-high heat.
Add ground beef and cook for approximately 5 minutes or till browned completely.
Transfer the beef in a bowl.
In a similar pan, melt 1 tablespoon of coconut oil on medium-high heat.
Add zucchini and bell peppers and stir fry for around 3-4 minutes.
Transfer the vegetables inside bowl with chicken.
In exactly the same pan, melt remaining coconut oil on medium heat.
Add garlic, ginger, turmeric and red chile and sauté for approximately 1-2 minutes.
Add chicken mixture, honey and coconut amino and increase the heat to high.
Cook, stirring occasionally for approximately 4-5 minutes or till sauce is nearly reduced.
Stir in remaining ingredients and take off from heat.
Nutrition:
Calories: 407 | Fat: 7g | Carbohydrates: 20g | Fiber: 13g | Protein: 36g

CHICKEN &VEGGIE CASSEROLE

Preparation time: 15 minutes
Cooking time: half an hour
Servings: 4
Ingredients
1/3 cup dijon mustard
1/3 cup organic honey
1 teaspoon dried basil
¼ teaspoon ground turmeric
1 teaspoon dried basil, crushed
Salt and freshly ground black pepper, to taste
1¾ pound chicken breasts
1 cup fresh white mushrooms, sliced
½ head broccoli, cut into small florets
Directions
Preheat the oven to 350 degrees f. Lightly, grease a baking dish.
In a bowl, mix together all ingredients except chicken, mushrooms and broccoli.
Arrange chicken in prepared baking dish and top with mushroom slices.
Place broccoli florets around chicken evenly.
Pour 1 / 2 of honey mixture over chicken and broccoli evenly.
Bake for approximately twenty minutes.
Now, coat the chicken with remaining sauce and bake for approximately 10 minutes.
Nutrition:
Calories: 427 | Fat: 9 g | Carbohydrates: 16g | Fiber: 7g| Protein: 35g

CHICKEN & CAULIFLOWER RICE CASSEROLE

Preparation time: fifteen minutes
Cooking time: an hour fifteen minutes
Servings: 8-10
Ingredients
2 tablespoons coconut oil, divided
3-pound bone-in chicken thighs and drumsticks
Salt and freshly ground black pepper, to taste
3 carrots, peeled and sliced
1 onion, chopped finely
2 garlic cloves, chopped finely
2 tablespoons fresh cinnamon, chopped finely
2 teaspoons ground cumin
1 teaspoon ground coriander
12 teaspoon ground cinnamon
½ teaspoon ground turmeric
1 teaspoon paprika
¼ teaspoon red pepper cayenne
1 (28-ounce) can diced tomatoes with liquid
1 red bell pepper, seeded and cut into thin strips
½ cup fresh parsley leaves, minced
Salt, to taste
1 head cauliflower, grated to some rice like consistency
1 lemon, sliced thinly
Directions
Preheat the oven to 375 degrees f.
In a large pan, melt 1 tablespoon of coconut oil high heat.
Add chicken pieces and cook for about 3-5 minutes per side or till golden brown.
Transfer the chicken in a plate.
In a similar pan, sauté the carrot, onion, garlic and ginger for about 4-5 minutes on medium heat.
Stir in spices and remaining coconut oil.
Add chicken, tomatoes, bell pepper, parsley and salt and simmer for approximately 3-5 minutes.
In the bottom of a 13x9-inch rectangular baking dish, spread the cauliflower rice evenly.
Place chicken mixture over cauliflower rice evenly and top with lemon slices.
With a foil paper, cover the baking dish and bake for approximately 35 minutes.
Uncover the baking dish and bake approximately 25 minutes.
Nutrition:
Calories: 412 | Fat: 12g | Carbohydrates: 23g | Fiber: 7g | Protein: 34g

CHICKEN MEATLOAF WITH VEGGIES

Preparation time: 20 minutes
Cooking time: 1-1¼ hours
Servings: 4
Ingredients
For meatloaf:
½ cup cooked chickpeas
2 egg whites
2½ teaspoons poultry seasoning
Salt and freshly ground black pepper, to taste
10-ounce lean ground chicken
1 cup red bell pepper, seeded and minced
1 cup celery stalk, minced
1/3 cup steel-cut oats
1 cup tomato puree, divided
2 tablespoons dried onion flakes, crushed
1 tablespoon prepared mustard
For veggies:
2-pounds summer squash, sliced
16-ounce frozen brussels sprouts
2 tablespoons extra-virgin extra virgin olive oil
Salt and freshly ground black pepper, to taste
Directions
Preheat the oven to 350 degrees f. Grease a 9x5-inch loaf pan.
In a mixer, add chickpeas, egg whites, poultry seasoning, salt and black pepper and pulse till smooth.
Transfer a combination in a large bowl.
Add chicken, veggies oats, ½ cup of tomato puree and onion flakes and mix till well combined.
Transfer the amalgamation into prepared loaf pan evenly.
With both hands, press, down the amalgamation slightly.
In another bowl mix together mustard and remaining tomato puree.
Place the mustard mixture over loaf pan evenly.
Bake approximately 1-1¼ hours or till desired doneness.
Meanwhile in a big pan of water, arrange a steamer basket.
Bring to a boil and set summer time squash i steamer basket.
Cover and steam approximately 10-12 minutes.
Drain well and aside.
Now, prepare the brussels sprouts according to package's directions.
In a big bowl, add veggies, oil, salt and black pepper and toss to coat well.
Serve the meatloaf with veggies.
Nutrition:
Calories: 420 | Fat: 9g | Carbohydrates: 21g | Fiber: 14g | Protein: 36g

ROASTED SPATCHCOCK CHICKEN	CREAMY MUSHROOM AND BROCCOLI CHICKEN
Preparation time: twenty or so minutes *Cooking time: 50 minutes* *Servings: 4-6* **Ingredients** *1 (4-pound) whole chicken* *1 (1-inch) piece fresh ginger, sliced* *4 garlic cloves, chopped* *1 small bunch fresh thyme* *Pinch of cayenne* *Salt and freshly ground black pepper, to taste* *¼ cup fresh lemon juice* *3 tablespoons extra virgin olive oil* **Directions** Arrange chicken, breast side down onto a large cutting board. With a kitchen shear, begin with thigh and cut along 1 side of backbone and turn chicken around. Now, cut along sleep issues and discard the backbone. Change the inside and open it like a book. Flatten the backbone firmly to flatten. In a food processor, add all ingredients except chicken and pulse till smooth. In a big baking dish, add the marinade mixture. Add chicken and coat with marinade generously. With a plastic wrap, cover the baking dish and refrigerate to marinate for overnight. Preheat the oven to 450 degrees f. Arrange a rack in a very roasting pan. Remove the chicken from refrigerator make onto rack over roasting pan, skin side down. Roast for about 50 minutes, turning once in the middle way. **Nutrition:** *Calories: 419	Fat: 14g	Carbohydrates: 28g |* *Fiber: 4g	Protein: 40g*	*Preparation time: 15 minutes* *Cooking time: 6 hours* *Servings: 6* **Ingredients** *1 10.5 ounce can of low-sodium cream of mushroom soup* *1 21 ounce can of low-sodium cream of chicken soup* *2 whole cooked chicken breasts, chopped or shredded* *2 cup milk* *1lb broccoli florets* *¼ teaspoon garlic powder* **Directions** Place all ingredients to a 5 quart or larger slow cooker and mix well. Cover and cook on low for 6 hours. Serve with potatoes, pasta, or rice. **Nutrition:** *Calories: 155	Fat: 2g	Carbohydrates: 19g |* *Fiber: 2g	Protein: 12g |Potassium 755mg* *|Sodium 35mg*

CHICKEN CURRY	APPLE & CINNAMON SPICED HONEY PORK LOIN
Preparation time: 10 minutes *Cooking time: 4 minutes* *Servings: 4* **Ingredients** *1lb skinless chicken breasts* *1 medium onion, thinly sliced* *1 15 ounce can chickpeas, drained and rinsed well* *2 medium sweet potatoes, peeled and diced* *½ cup light coconut milk* *½ cup chicken stock (see recipe)* *1 15ounce can sodium-free tomato sauce* *2 tablespoon curry powder* *1 teaspoon low-sodium salt* *½ cayenne powder* *1 cup green peas* *2 tablespoon lemon juice* **Directions** Place the chicken breasts, onion, chickpeas, and sweet potatoes into a 4 to 6-quart slow cooker. Mix the coconut milk, chicken stock, tomato sauce, curry powder, salt, and cayenne together and pour into the slow cooker, stirring to coat well. Cover and cook on low for 8 hours or high for 4 hours. Stir in the peas and lemon juice 5 minutes before serving. **Nutrition:** *Calories: 302	Fat: 5g	Carbohydrates: 43g	Fiber: 9g	Protein: 24g |Potassium 573mg |Sodium 800mg*	*Preparation time: 20 minutes* *Cooking time: 6 hours* *Servings: 6* **Ingredients** *1 2-3lb boneless pork loin roast* *½ teaspoon low-sodium salt* *¼ teaspoon pepper* *1 tablespoon canola oil* *3 medium apples, peeled and sliced* *¼ cup honey* *1 small red onion, halved and sliced* *1 tablespoon ground cinnamon* **Directions** Season the pork with salt and pepper. Heat the oil in a skillet and brown the pork on all sides. Arrange half the apples in the base of a 4 to 6-quart slow cooker. Top with the honey and remaining apples. Sprinkle with cinnamon and cover. Cover and cook on low for 6-8 hours until the meat is tender. **Nutrition:** *Calories: 290	Fat: 10 g	Carbohydrates: 19g	Fiber: 2g	Protein: 29g |Potassium 789mg |Sodium 22mg*

LEMON & HERB TURKEY BREASTS

Preparation time: 25 minutes
Cooking time: 3 1/2 hours
Servings: 12

Ingredients

1 can (14-1/2 ounces) chicken broth
1/2 cup lemon juice
1/4 cup packed brown sugar
1/4 cup fresh sage
1/4 cup fresh thyme leaves
1/4 cup lime juice
1/4 cup cider vinegar
1/4 cup olive oil
1 envelope low-sodium onion soup mix
2 tablespoon dijon mustard
1 tablespoon fresh marjoram, minced
1 teaspoon paprika
1 teaspoon garlic powder
1 teaspoon pepper
½ teaspoon low-sodium salt
2 2lb boneless skinless turkey breast halves

Directions

Make a marinade by blending all the ingredients in a blender.
Pour over the turkey and leave overnight.
Place the turkey and marinade in a 4 to 6-quart slow cooker and cover.
Cover and cook on high for 3-1/2 to 4-1/2 hours or until a thermometer reads 165°.

Nutrition:

Calories: 219 | Fat: 5g | Carbohydrates: 3g | Fiber: 0g | Protein: 36g | Potassium 576mg | Sodium 484mg

BEEF CHIMICHANGAS

Preparation time: 10minutes
Cooking time: 10-12 hours
Servings: 16

Ingredients

Shredded beef
3lb boneless beef chuck roast, fat trimmed away
3 tablespoon low-sodium taco seasoning mix
1 10ounce canned low-sodium diced tomatoes
6ounce canned diced green chilies with the juice
3 garlic cloves, minced
To serve
16 medium flour tortillas
Sodium-free refried beans
Mexican rice, sour cream, cheddar cheese
Guacamole, salsa, lettuce

Directions

Arrange the beef in a 5-quart or larger slow cooker.
Sprinkle over taco seasoning and coat well.
Add tomatoes and garlic and cover.
Cook on low for 10 to 12 hours.
When cooked remove the beef and shred.
Make burritos out of the shredded beef, refried beans, mexican rice, and cheese.
Bake for 10 minutes at 350° f until brown.
Serve with salsa, lettuce, and guacamole.

Nutrition:

Calories: 249 | Fat: 18g | Carbohydrates: 3g | Fiber: 5g | Protein: 33g | Potassium 633mg | Sodium 457mg

MEAT LOAF

Preparation time: 5 minutes
Cooking time: 5-6 hours
Servings: 6

Ingredients

2-pound lean ground beef
2 whole eggs, beaten
¾ cup milk
¾ cup breadcrumbs
½ cup chicken broth (see recipe)
¼ cup onion, finely diced
3 garlic cloves, minced
1 teaspoon low-sodium salt
¼ teaspoon freshly ground black pepper
¼ cup low sodium chili sauce
Nonstick spray

Directions

Mix the beaten eggs, milk, oatmeal, spices, onion, garlic, and chicken broth until well combined.
Mix in the beef and place in a 5-quart or larger slow cooker, sprayed with nonstick spray.
Cover and cook on low for 5 to 6 hours.
Serve with low-sodium ketchup.

Nutrition:

Calories: 280 | Fat: 10g | Carbohydrates: 9g | Fiber: 1g | Protein: 12g |Potassium 648mg |Sodium 325mg

Chapter 17: Meat

LAMB WITH PRUNES

Preparation Time: 15 minutes
Cooking Time: 2 hours and 40 minutes
Servings: 4-6
Ingredients
3 tablespoons coconut oil
2 onions, chopped finely
1 (1-inch) piece fresh ginger, minced
3 garlic cloves, minced
½ teaspoon ground turmeric
2 ½ pound lamb shoulder, trimmed and cubed into 3-inch size
Salt and freshly ground black pepper, to taste
½ teaspoon saffron threads, crumbled
1 cinnamon stick
3 cups water
1 cup runes, pitted and halved
Directions
In a big pan, melt coconut oil on medium heat.
Add onions, ginger, garlic cloves and turmeric and sauté for about 3-5 minutes.
Sprinkle the lamb with salt and black pepper evenly.
In the pan, add lamb and saffron threads and cook for approximately 4-5 minutes.
Add cinnamon stick and water and produce to some boil on high heat.
Reduce the temperature to low and simmer, covered for around 1½-120 minutes or till desired doneness of lamb.
Stir in prunes and simmer for approximately 20-a half-hour.
Remove cinnamon stick and serve hot.
Nutrition:
Calories: 393 | Fat: 12g | Carbohydrates: 10g | Fiber: 4g | Protein: 36g

ROAST BEEF

Preparation Time: 25 minutes
Cooking Time: 55 minutes
Servings: 3
Ingredients
Quality rump or sirloin tip roast
Direction:
Place in roasting pan o n a shallow rack
Season with pepper and herbs
Insert meat thermometer in the center or thickest part of the roast
Roast to the desired degree of doneness
After removing from over for about 15 minutes let it chill
In the end the roast should be moister than well done.
Nutrition:
Calories: 158 | Fat: 6g | Carbohydrates: 0g | Protein: 24g |Potassium 328mg |Sodium 55mg | Phosphorus 206mg

BEEF BROCHETTES	COUNTRY FRIED STEAK
Preparation Time: 20 minutes *Cooking Time: 1 hour* *Servings: 1* **Ingredients** *1 ½ cups pineapple chunks* *1 sliced large onion* *2 pounds thick steak* *1 sliced medium bell pepper* *1 bay leaf* *¼ cup vegetable oil* *½ cup lemon juice* *2 crushed garlic cloves* **Directions** Cut beef cubes and place in a plastic bag Combine marinade ingredients in small bowl Mix and pour over beef cubes Seal the bag and refrigerate for 3 to 5 hours Divide ingredients onion, beef cube, green pepper, pineapple Grill about 9 minutes each side **Nutrition:** *Calories: 304	Fat: 15g	Carbohydrates: 11g |* *Protein: 35g |Potassium 388mg |Sodium 70mg |* *Phosphorus 264mg*	*Preparation Time: 10 minutes* *Cooking Time: 1 hour and 40 minutes* *Servings: 3* **Ingredients** *1 large onion* *½ cup flour* *3 tablespoons. vegetable oil* *¼ teaspoon pepper* *1½ pounds round steak* *½ teaspoon paprika* **Directions** Trim excess fat from steak Cut into small pieces Combine flour, paprika and pepper and mix together Preheat skillet with oil Cook steak on both sides When the color of steak is brown remove to a platter Add water (150 ml) and stir around the skillet Return browned steak to skillet, if necessary, add water again so that bottom side of steak does not stick **Nutrition:** *Calories: 248	Fat: 10g	Carbohydrates: 5g |* *Protein: 30g |Potassium 338mg |Sodium 60mg |* *Phosphorus 190mg*

BEEF POT ROAST	HOMEMADE BURGERS
Preparation Time: 20 minutes *Cooking Time: 1 hour* *Servings: 3* **Ingredients** *Round bone roast* *2 - 4 pounds chuck roast* **Direction**: Trim off excess fat Place a tablespoon of oil in a large skillet and heat to medium Roll pot roast in flour and brown on all sides in a hot skillet After the meat gets a brown color, reduce heat to low Season with pepper and herbs and add ½ cup of water Cook slowly for 1½ hours or until it looks ready **Nutrition:** *Calories: 157 | Fat: 13g | Carbohydrates: 0g | Protein: 24g |Potassium 328mg |Sodium 50mg | Phosphorus 204mg*	*Preparation Time: 10 minutes* *Cooking Time: 20 minutes* *Servings: 2* **Ingredients** *4 ounce lean 100% ground beef* *1 teaspoon black pepper* *1 garlic clove, minced* *1 teaspoon olive oil* *1/4 cup onion, finely diced* *1 tablespoon balsamic vinegar* *1/2ounce brie cheese, crumbled* *1 teaspoon mustard* **Directions** Season ground beef with pepper and then mix in minced garlic. Form burger shapes with the ground beef using the palms of your hands. Heat a skillet on a medium to high heat, and then add the oil. Sauté the onions for 5-10 minutes until browned. Then add the balsamic vinegar and sauté for another 5 minutes. Remove and set aside. Add the burgers to the pan and heat on the same heat for 5-6 minutes before flipping and heating for a further 5-6 minutes until cooked through. Spread the mustard onto each burger. Crumble the brie cheese over each burger and serve! Try with a crunchy side salad! Tip: If using fresh beef and not defrosted, prepare double the ingredients and freeze burgers in plastic wrap (after cooling) for up to 1 month. Thoroughly defrost before heating through completely in the oven to serve. **Nutrition:** *Calories: 178 | Fat: 10g | Carbohydrates: 4g | Protein: 16g |Potassium 272mg |Sodium 273mg | Phosphorus 147mg*

SLOW-COOKED BEEF BRISKET

Preparation Time: 10 minutes
Cooking Time: 3 hours and 30 minutes
Servings: 6
Ingredients
10-ounce chuck roast
1 onion, sliced
1 cup carrots, peeled and sliced
1 tablespoon mustard
1 tablespoon thyme (fresh or dried)
1 tablespoon rosemary (fresh or dried)
2 garlic cloves
2 tablespoon extra-virgin olive oil
1 teaspoon black pepper
1 cup homemade chicken stock (p.52)
1 cup water
Directions
Preheat oven to 300°f/150°c/Gas Mark 2.
Trim any fat from the beef and soak vegetables in warm water.
Make a paste by mixing together the mustard, thyme, rosemary, and garlic, before mixing in the oil and pepper.
Combine this mix with the stock.
Pour the mixture over the beef into an oven proof baking dish.
Place the vegetables onto the bottom of the baking dish with the beef.
Cover and roast for 3 hours, or until tender.
Uncover the dish and continue to cook for 30 minutes in the oven.
Serve hot!
Nutrition:
Calories: 151 | Fat: 7g | Carbohydrates: 7g | Protein: 15g |Potassium 344mg |Sodium 279mg | Phosphorus 144mg

PORK SOUVLAKI

Preparation time: 20 minutes
Cooking time: 12 minutes
Servings: 8
Ingredients
Olive oil – 3 tablespoons
Lemon juice – 2 tablespoons
Minced garlic – 1 teaspoon
Chopped fresh oregano – 1 tablespoon
Ground black pepper – ¼ teaspoon
Pork leg – 1 pound, cut in 2-inch cubes
Directions
In a bowl, stir together the lemon juice, olive oil, garlic, oregano, and pepper.
Add the pork cubes and toss to coat.
Place the bowl in the refrigerator, covered, for 2 hours to marinate.
Thread the pork chunks onto 8 wooden skewers that have been soaked in water.
Preheat the barbecue to medium-high heat.
Grill the pork skewers for about 12 minutes, turning once, until just cooked through but still juicy.
Nutrition:
Calories: 95 | Fat: 4g | Carbohydrates: 0g | Protein: 13g |Potassium 230mg |Sodium 29mg | Phosphorus 125mg

OPEN-FACED BEEF STIR-UP	**GRILLED STEAK WITH CUCUMBER SALSA**
Preparation time: 10 minutes *Cooking time: 10 minutes* *Servings: 6* **Ingredients** *95% Lean ground beef – ½ pound* *Chopped sweet onion – ½ cup* *Shredded cabbage – ½ cup* *Herb pesto – ¼ cup* *Hamburger buns – 6, bottom halves only* **Directions** Sauté the beef and onion for 6 minutes or until beef is cooked. Add the cabbage and sauté for 3 minutes more. Stir in pesto and heat for 1 minute. Divide the beef mixture into 6 portions and serve each on the bottom half of a hamburger bun, open-face. **Nutrition:** *Calories: 120 | Fat: 3g | Protein: 11g |Potassium 198mg |Sodium 134mg | Phosphorus 106mg*	*Preparation time: 20 minutes* *Cooking time: 15 minutes* *Servings: 4* **Ingredients** **For the salsa** *Chopped English cucumber - 1 cup* *Boiled and diced red bell pepper – ¼ cup* *Scallion – 1, both green and white parts, chopped* *Chopped fresh cilantro – 2 tablespoons* *Juice of 1 lime* **For the steak** *Beef tenderloin steaks – 4 (3-ounce), room temperature* *Olive oil* *Freshly ground black pepper* **Directions** To make the salsa, in a bowl combine the lime juice, cilantro, scallion, bell pepper, and cucumber. Set aside. To make the steak: Preheat a barbecue to medium heat. Rub the steaks all over with oil and season with pepper. Grill the steaks for about 5 minutes per side for medium-rare, or until the desired state. Serve the steaks topped with salsa. **Nutrition:** *Calories: 130 | Fat: 6g | Carbohydrates: 1g | Protein: 19g |Potassium 272mg |Sodium 39mg | Phosphorus 186mg*

BEEF BRISKET

Preparation time: 10 minutes
Cooking time: 3 ½ hours
Servings: 6
Ingredients
Chuck roast – 12 ounces trimmed
Garlic – 2 cloves
Thyme – 1 tablespoon
Rosemary – tablespoon
Mustard - 1 tablespoon
Extra virgin olive oil – ¼ cup
Black pepper – 1 teaspoon
Onion – 1, diced
Carrots – 1 cup, peeled and sliced
Low salt stock – 2 cups

Directions
Preheat the oven to 300F.
Soak vegetables in warm water.
Make a paste by mixing together the thyme, mustard, rosemary, and garlic. Then mix in the oil and pepper.
Add the beef to the dish.
Pour the mixture over the beef into a dish.
Place the vegetables onto the bottom of the baking dish around the beef.
Cover and roast for 3 hours, or until tender.
Uncover the dish and continue to cook for 30 minutes in the oven.
Serve.
Nutrition:
Calories: 303 | Fat: 25g | Carbohydrates: 7g | Protein: 18g |Potassium 246mg |Sodium 44mg | Phosphorus 376mg

APRICOT AND LAMB TAGINE

Preparation time: 10 minutes
Cooking time: 1 to 1 ½ hours
Servings: 2
Ingredients
Extra virgin olive oil – 1 tablespoon
Lean lamb fillets – 2, cubed
Onion – 1, diced
Homemade chicken stock – 4 cups
Cumin – 1 teaspoon
Turmeric – 1 teaspoon
Curry powder – 1 teaspoon
Dried rosemary – 1 teaspoon
Chopped parsley – 1 teaspoon
Canned apricots – ½ cup, juices drained and apricots rinsed

Directions
Heat the olive oil in a pot.
Add lamb to the pot and cook for 5 minutes or until browned.
Remove lamb and set aside.
Add the chopped onion to the pot and sauté for 5 minutes, or until starting to soften.
Sprinkle with cumin, curry powder, and turmeric over the onions and continue to stir for 4 to 5 minutes.
Now add the lamb back into the pot with the chicken stock and rosemary.
Cover the pot and leave to simmer on a low heat for 1 to 1.5 hours or until the lamb is tender and fully cooked through.
Add the apricots 15 minutes before the end of the cooking time.
Garnish with parsley and serve.
Nutrition:
Calories: 193 | Fat: 12g | Carbohydrates: 9g | Protein: 20g |Potassium 156mg |Sodium 105mg | Phosphorus 170mg

LAMB SHOULDER WITH ZUCCHINI AND EGGPLANT

Preparation time: 10 minutes
Cooking time: 4 to 5 hours
Servings: 2

Ingredients

Lean lamb shoulder – 6 ounces
Zucchinis – 2, cubed
Eggplant – 1, cubed
Black pepper – 1 teaspoon
Extra virgin olive oil – 2 tablespoons
Basil – 1 tablespoon
Oregano – 1 tablespoon
Garlic – 2 cloves, chopped

Directions

Preheat the oven to its highest setting.

Soak the vegetables in warm water.

Trim any fat from the lamb shoulder.

Rub the lamb with 1 tablespoon olive oil, pepper, and herbs.

Line a baking tray with the rest of the olive oil, garlic, zucchini, and eggplant.

Add the lamb shoulder and cover with foil.

Turn the oven down to 325F and add the dish into the oven.

Cook for 4 to 5 hours, remove and rest.

Slice the lamb and then serve with the vegetables.

Nutrition:

Calories: 478 | Fat: 31g | Carbohydrates: 13g | Protein: 33g |Potassium 414mg |Sodium 84mg | Phosphorus 197mg

Chapter 18: Desserts

DESSERT COCKTAIL

Preparation time: 1 minutes
Cooking time: 0 minute
Servings: 4
Ingredients
1 cup of cranberry juice
1 cup of fresh ripe strawberries, washed and hull removed
2 tablespoon of lime juice
¼ cup of white sugar
8 ice cubes
Directions
Combine all the ingredients in a blender until smooth and creamy.
Pour the liquid into chilled tall glasses and serve cold.
Nutrition:
Calories: 92 | Fat: 0.17g | Carbohydrates: 23.5 | Protein: 0.5g |Potassium 103.78mg |Sodium 3.62mg | Phosphorus 17.86mg | Fiber0.84g

BAKED EGG CUSTARD

Preparation time: 15 minutes
Cooking time: 30 minutes
Servings: 4
Ingredients
2 medium eggs, at room temperature
¼ cup of semi-skimmed milk
3 tablespoons of white sugar
½ teaspoon of nutmeg
1 teaspoon of vanilla extract
Directions
Preheat your oven at 375 f/180c
Mix all the ingredients in a mixing bowl and beat with a hand mixer for a few seconds until creamy and uniform.
Pour the mixture into lightly greased muffin tins.
Bake for 25-30 minutes or until the knife, you place inside, comes out clean.

Nutrition:
Calories: 96.56 | Fat: 2.91g | Carbohydrates: 10.5g | Protein: 3.5g |Potassium 58.19mg |Sodium 37.75mg | Phosphorus 58.76mg | Fiber 0.06g

GUMDROP COOKIES

Preparation time: 15 minutes
Cooking time: 12 minutes
Servings: 25
Ingredients
½ cup of spreadable unsalted butter
1 medium egg
1 cup of brown sugar
1 ⅔ cups of all-purpose flour, sifted
¼ cup of milk
1 teaspoon vanilla
1 teaspoon of baking powder
15 large gumdrops, chopped finely
Directions
Preheat the oven at 400f/195c.
Combine the sugar, butter and egg until creamy.
Add the milk and vanilla and stir well.
Combine the flour with the baking powder in a different bowl. Incorporate to the sugar, butter mixture, and stir.
Add the gumdrops and place the mixture in the fridge for half an hour.
Drop the dough with tablespoonful into a lightly greased baking or cookie sheet.
Bake for 10-12 minutes or until golden brown in color.
Nutrition:
Calories: 102.17 | Fat: 4g | Carbohydrates: 16.5g | Protein: 0.86g |Potassium 45mg |Sodium 23.42mg | Phosphorus 32.15mg | Fiber 0.13g

POUND CAKE WITH PINEAPPLE

Preparation time: 10 minutes
Cooking time: 50 minutes
Servings: 24
Ingredients
3 cups of all-purpose flour, sifted
3 cups of sugar
1 ½ cups of butter
6 whole eggs and 3 egg whites
1 teaspoon of vanilla extract
1 10. Ounce can of pineapple chunks, rinsed and crushed (keep juice aside).
For glaze:
1 cup of sugar
1 stick of unsalted butter or margarine
Reserved juice from the pineapple

Directions
Preheat the oven at 350f/180c.
Beat the sugar and the butter with a hand mixer until creamy and smooth.
Slowly add the eggs (one or two every time) and stir well after pouring each egg.
Add the vanilla extract, follow up with the flour and stir well.
Add the drained and chopped pineapple.
Pour the mixture into a greased cake tin and bake for 45-50 minutes.
In a small saucepan, combine the sugar with the butter and pineapple juice. Stir every few seconds and bring to boil. Cook until you get a creamy to thick glaze consistency.
Pour the glaze over the cake while still hot.
Let cook for at least 10 seconds and serve.
Nutrition:
Calories: 407 | Fat: 16g | Carbohydrates: 79g | Protein: 4.25g |Potassium 180mg |Sodium 118mg | Phosphorus 66mg | Fiber 2.25g

APPLE CRUNCH PIE	SPICED PEACHES
Preparation time: 10 minutes *Cooking time: 35 minutes* *Servings: 8* **Ingredients** *4 large tart apples, peeled, seeded and sliced* *½ cup of white all-purpose flour* *⅓ cup margarine* *1 cup of sugar* *¾ cup of rolled oat flakes* *½ teaspoon of ground nutmeg* **Directions** Preheat the oven to 375f/180c. Place the apples over a lightly greased square pan (around 7 inches). Mix the rest of the ingredients in a medium bowl with and spread the batter over the apples. Bake for 30-35 minutes or until the top crust has gotten golden brown. Serve hot. **Nutrition:** *Calories: 262 | Fat: 8g | Carbohydrates: 47g | Protein: 1.5g |Potassium 123mg |Sodium 81mg | Phosphorus 35mg | Fiber 2.81g*	*Preparation time: 5 minutes* *Cooking time: 10 minutes* *Servings: 2* **Ingredients** *Canned peaches with juices – 1 cup* *Cornstarch – ½ teaspoon* *Ground cloves – 1 teaspoon* *Ground cinnamon – 1 teaspoon* *Ground nutmeg – 1 teaspoon* *Zest of ½ lemon* *Water – ½ cup* **Directions** Drain peaches. Combine cinnamon, cornstarch, nutmeg, ground cloves, and lemon zest in a pan on the stove. Heat on a medium heat and add peaches. Bring to a boil, reduce the heat and simmer for 10 minutes. Serve. **Nutrition:** *Calories: 70 | Fat: 0g | Protein: 1g |Potassium 176mg |Sodium 3mg | Phosphorus 23mg*

PUMPKIN CHEESECAKE BAR	BLUEBERRY MINI MUFFINS

PUMPKIN CHEESECAKE BAR

Preparation time: 10 minutes
Cooking time: 50 minutes
Servings: 4
Ingredients
Unsalted butter – 2 ½ tablespoons.
Cream cheese – 4 ounces
All-purpose white flour – ½ cup
Golden brown sugar – 3 tablespoons.
Granulated sugar – ¼ cup
Pureed pumpkin – ½ cup
Egg whites - 2
Ground cinnamon – 1 teaspoon
Ground nutmeg – 1 teaspoon
Vanilla extract – 1 teaspoon

Directions
Preheat the oven to 350f.
Mix flour and brown sugar in a bowl.
Mix in the butter to form 'breadcrumbs.
Place ¾ of this mixture in a dish.
Bake in the oven for 15 minutes. Remove and cool.
Lightly whisk the egg and fold in the cream cheese, sugar, pumpkin, cinnamon, nutmeg and vanilla until smooth.
Pour this mixture over the oven-baked base and sprinkle with the rest of the breadcrumbs from earlier.
Bake in the oven for 30 to 35 minutes more.
Cool, slice and serve.
Nutrition:
Calories: 248 | Fat: 13g | Protein: 4g |Potassium 96mg |Sodium 146mg | Phosphorus 67mg | Carbohydrates: 33g

BLUEBERRY MINI MUFFINS

Preparation time: 10 minutes
Cooking time: 35 minutes
Servings: 4
Ingredients
Egg whites – 3
All-purpose white flour – ¼ cup
Coconut flour – 1 tablespoon
Baking soda – 1 teaspoon
Nutmeg – 1 tablespoon grated
Vanilla extract – 1 teaspoon
Stevia – 1 teaspoon
Fresh blueberries – ¼ cup
Directions
Preheat the oven to 325f.
Mix all the ingredients in a bowl.
Divide the batter into 4 and spoon into a lightly oiled muffin tin.
Bake in the oven for 15 to 20 minutes or until cooked through.
Cool and serve.
Nutrition:
Calories: 62 | Fat: 0 | Protein: 4g |Potassium 65mg | Sodium 62mg | Phosphorus 103mg | Carbohydrates: 9g

VANILLA CUSTARD	CHOCOLATE CHIP COOKIES
Preparation time: 7 minutes *Cooking time: 10 minutes* *Servings: 10* **Ingredients** *Egg – 1* *Vanilla – 1/8 teaspoon* *Nutmeg – 1/8 teaspoon* *Almond milk – ½ cup* *Stevia - 2 tablespoon* **Directions** Scald the milk then let it cool slightly. Break the egg into a bowl and beat it with the nutmeg. Add the scalded milk, the vanilla, and the sweetener to taste. Mix well. Place the bowl in a baking pan filled with ½ deep of water. Bake for 30 minutes at 325f. Serve. **Nutrition:** *Calories: 167 | Fat: 9g | Protein: 10g |Potassium 249mg |Sodium 124mg | Phosphorus 205mg | Carbohydrates: 11g*	*Preparation time: 7 minutes* *Cooking time: 10 minutes* *Servings: 10* **Ingredients** *Semi-sweet chocolate chips – ½ cup* *Baking soda – ½ teaspoon* *Vanilla – ½ teaspoon* *Egg – 1* *Flour – 1 cup* *Margarine – ½ cup* *Stevia – 4 teaspoons* **Directions** Sift the dry ingredients. Cream the margarine, stevia, vanilla and egg with a whisk. Add flour mixture and beat well. Stir in the chocolate chips, then drop teaspoonfuls of the mixture over a greased baking sheet. Bake the cookies for about 10 minutes at 375f. Cool and serve. **Nutrition:** *Calories: 106.2 | Fat: 7g | Protein: 1.5g |Potassium 28mg |Sodium 98mg | Phosphorus 19mg | Carbohydrates: 8.9g*

LEMON MOUSSE

Preparation time: 10 + chill time
Cooking time: 10 minutes
Servings: 4

Ingredients

1 cup coconut cream
8 ounces cream cheese, soft
¼ cup fresh lemon juice
3 pinches salt
1 teaspoon lemon liquid stevia

Directions

Preheat your oven to 350 °f
Grease a ramekin with butter
Beat cream, cream cheese, fresh lemon juice, salt and lemon liquid stevia in a mixer
Pour batter into ramekin
Bake for 10 minutes, then transfer the mousse to a serving glass
Let it chill for 2 hours and serve
Enjoy!

Nutrition:

Calories: 395 | Fat: 31g | Protein: 5g | Carbohydrates: 3g

JALAPENO CRISP

Preparation time: 10 minutes
Cooking time: 1 hour 15 minutes
Servings: 20

Ingredients

1 cup sesame seeds
1 cup sunflower seeds
1 cup flaxseeds
½ cup hulled hemp seeds
3 tablespoons psyllium husk
1 teaspoon salt
1 teaspoon baking powder
2 cups of water

Directions

Pre-heat your oven to 350 °f
Take your blender and add seeds, baking powder, salt, and psyllium husk
Blend well until a sand-like texture appears
Stir in water and mix until a batter form
Allow the batter to rest for 10 minutes until a dough-like thick mixture forms
Pour the dough onto a cookie sheet lined with parchment paper
Spread it evenly, making sure that it has a thickness of ¼ inch thick all around
Bake for 75 minutes in your oven
Remove and cut into 20 spices
Allow them to cool for 30 minutes and enjoy!

Nutrition:

Calories: 156 | Fat: 13g | Protein: 5g | Carbohydrates: 2g

RASPBERRY POPSICLE	EASY FUDGE
Preparation time: 2 hours *Cooking time: 15 minutes* *Servings: 4* **Ingredients** *1 ½ cups raspberries* *2 cups of water* **Directions** Take a pan and fill it up with water Add raspberries Place it over medium heat and bring to water to a boil Reduce the heat and simmer for 15 minutes Remove heat and pour the mix into popsicle molds Add a popsicle stick and let it chill for 2 hours Serve and enjoy! **Nutrition:** Calories: 58 | Fat: 0.4g | Protein: 1.4g | Carbohydrates: 0g	*Preparation time: 15 minutes + chill time* *Cooking time: 5 minutes* *Servings: 25* **Ingredients** *1 ¾ cups of coconut butter* *1 cup pumpkin puree* *1 teaspoon ground cinnamon* *¼ teaspoon ground nutmeg* *1 tablespoon coconut oil* **Directions** Take an 8x8 inch square baking pan and line it with aluminum foil Take a spoon and scoop out the coconut butter into a heated pan and allow the butter to melt Keep stirring well and remove from the heat once fully melted Add spices and pumpkin and keep straining until you have a grain-like texture Add coconut oil and keep stirring to incorporate everything Scoop the mixture into your baking pan and evenly distribute it Place wax paper on top of the mixture and press gently to straighten the top Remove the paper and discard Allow it to chill for 1-2 hours Once chilled, take it out and slice it up into pieces Enjoy! **Nutrition:** Calories: 120 | Fat: 10g | Protein: 1.2g | Carbohydrates: 5g

COCONUT LOAF

Preparation time: 15 minutes
Cooking time: 40 minutes
Servings: 4
Ingredients
1 ½ tablespoons coconut flour
¼ teaspoon baking powder
1/8 teaspoon salt
1 tablespoon coconut oil, melted
1 whole egg
Directions
Preheat your oven to 350 °f
Add coconut flour, baking powder, salt
Add coconut oil, eggs and stir well until mixed
Leave the batter for several minutes
Pour half the batter onto the baking pan
Spread it to form a circle, repeat with remaining batter
Bake in the oven for 10 minutes
Once a golden-brown texture comes, let it cool and serve
Enjoy!
Nutrition:
Calories: 297 | Fat: 14 | Protein: 15g |
Carbohydrates: 15g

Conclusion

Renal diet may seem restricting for many, but in reality, there is plenty of low-sodium, low-phosphorus, and low-potassium options to try out and we have proven it with this recipe book.

Keep in mind that we have included roughly the levels of all these minerals in every recipe separately and therefore, you will have to calculate the total amounts you consume each day with all your daily meals.

Kidney disease now ranks as the 18th deadliest condition in the world. In the United States alone, it is reported that over 600,000 Americans succumb to kidney failure.

These stats are alarming, which is why, it is necessary to take proper care of your kidneys, starting with a kidney-friendly diet.

In this eBook, you will learn Direction create dishes that are healthy, delicious and easy on your kidneys.

These recipes are ideal whether you have been diagnosed with a kidney problem or you want to prevent any kidney issue.

With regards to your wellbeing and health, it's a smart thought to see your doctor as frequently as conceivable to ensure you don't run into preventable issues that you needn't get. The kidneys are your body's toxin channel (just like the liver), cleaning the blood of remote substances and toxins that are discharged from things like preservatives in food & other toxins.

The moment you eat boldly and fill your body with toxins, food, beverages (liquor or alcohol, for example). In general, your body will also convert a number of things that appear to be benign, until your organs convert them to things like formaldehyde, due to a synthetic response and the transformation phase.

One such case is a large proportion of dietary sugars used in diet sodas - for example, aspartame is converted to formaldehyde in the body.These toxins must be expelled or they can prompt ailment, renal (kidney) failure, malignant growth, & various other painful problems.

This isn't a condition that occurs without any forethought it is a dynamic issue and in that it very well may be both found early and treated, diet changed, and settling what is causing the issue is conceivable. It's conceivable to have partial renal failure yet, as a rule; it requires some time (or downright awful diet for a short time) to arrive at absolute renal failure. You would prefer not to reach total renal failure since this will require standard dialysis treatments to save your life.

Dialysis treatments explicitly clean the blood of waste and toxins in the blood utilizing a machine in light of the fact that your body can no longer carry out the responsibility. Without treatments, you could die a very painful death. Renal failure can be the consequence of long haul diabetes, hypertension, unreliable diet, and can stem from other health concerns.

A renal diet is tied in with directing the intake of protein and phosphorus in your eating routine. Restricting your sodium intake is likewise significant. By controlling these two variables you can control the vast majority of the toxins/waste made by your body and thus this enables your kidney to 100% function. In the event that you get this early enough and truly moderate your diets with extraordinary consideration, you could avert all-out renal failure. In the event that you get this early, you can take out the issue completely.

Generally, most experts suggest up to 2700 mg of potassium and phosphorus per day for patients at the first two stages of renal disease while those at a more advanced stage should aim to consume up to 2000mg of these two minerals (each) per day to avoid dialysis.

Don't forget to do regular doctor check-ups to monitor your progress.

CPSIA information can be obtained
at www.ICGtesting.com
Printed in the USA
LVHW101158010221
677999LV00009B/210